Mediterranean Diet For Beginners 2020

Step by Step Practical Guide For Beginners to Lose Weight, Be Long-Lived and Live in Health. Simple and Fast Recipes With a 21-Day Action Plan.

Elisa Rossi

or indirect, that are incurred as a result of the use of the information contained within this document, including, but not limited to, errors, omissions, or inaccuracies.

Thanks for choosing this book, make sure to leave a short review on Amazon if you enjoy it. I'd really love to hear your thoughts.

Summary

Introduction

A major part of any culture, region, or ethnic group is the food they indulge in. Whether you travel locally or abroad, you will find the people you meet here or there take great pride in the culinary treats that are standards for them. Food is a major part of our lives and oftentimes the catalyst of any great gathering or event. We love the food we eat, and also believe our local flavors are the best, better than any other. The meals we eat not only satisfy our cravings, but also provide us the nutrients we need. Without sustenance, we cannot live, nor can we fully enjoy life.

It makes sense then that food is a major part of our health and well-being. Unfortunately, many of the things we intake are not always the best for us. In many cases, we simply eat for the sake of taste, and don't have a second thought on how it impacts our health. If this continues for too long, then we face the possibility of severe health issues. What if there are options that provide a tasty meal that is also good for you? You would be describing the Mediterranean diet. This diet is diverse as it encompasses a wide variety of ingredients and food groups that are dense in nutrients. The meals are flavorful, and the ingredients will make you feel good.

With this book, an in-depth description tells you what the Mediterranean diet is, what it encompasses, and its various health benefits. I have compiled a number of detailed recipes for meal plans you can make your own. I have also given you tips on how to transition to the Mediterranean diet, including a 21-day meal plan. By the end of this book, you will have a new outlook on the idea of dieting and how to make it work for you.

When you introduce the Mediterranean diet into your meals and pair it with a healthy lifestyle, the results can change your life. You will notice a change in the way you feel, increased energy, and a regimen in place to fight off chronic illness. You will have all the information you need to understand how to make the most of your daily meals.

Chapter 1: What Is the Mediterranean Diet

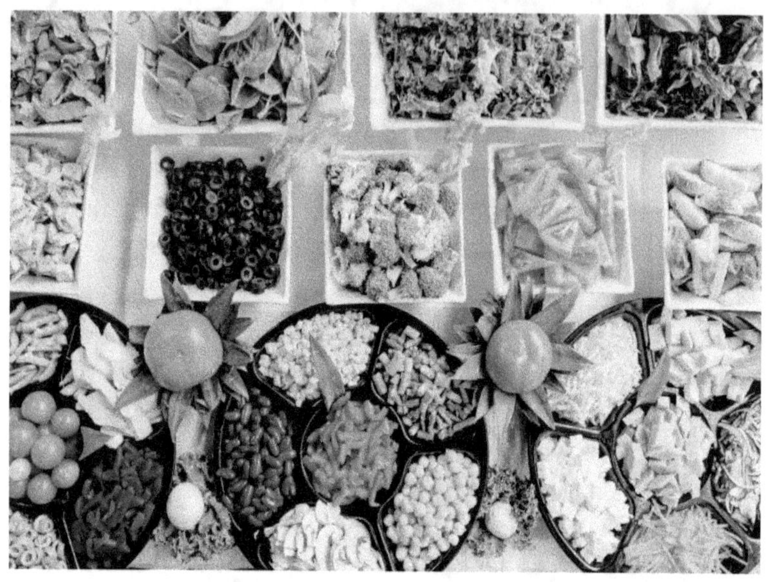

Food is a major staple in our lives. We cannot live without it, and for some, food is nothing more than sustenance. They eat to live as food is fuel. For others, it is a way of life. It is part of their culture and who they are. It is the main attraction of social events or gatherings, and every region in the world takes pride in their cuisine. It is what people turn to in some of their darkest times.

The Mediterranean diet originates from the region that surrounds the Mediterranean Sea in Europe. It encompasses the traditional cuisine from countries like Greece, Italy, France, Egypt, and Israel. There are over 20 countries considered as part of the Mediterranean, and each place has its own unique twist, supplying us with a wide variety of recipes. However, what does not change is the flavor and health benefits of the cuisines. In many respects, the ingredients are just used in a different manner. We will discuss these benefits in a later chapter.

The Mediterranean diet utilizes a diverse amount of healthy food groups and ingredients. The major food groups include:

- A wide variety of fruits and vegetables. Some common fruits and vegetables are berries, watermelons, apples, oranges, grapes. tomatoes, olives, broccoli, cauliflower, potatoes, and radishes.
- Whole grains and nuts, different from refined grains in that they hold onto all of their nutritional value. For example, barley, buckwheat, whole oats, quinoa, and whole wheat are considered whole grains. Healthy nuts include almonds, walnuts, pistachios, and pecans.
- Fatty fishes like tuna, salmon, trout, and mackerel are a major source of protein and omega-3 fatty acids. A major rule is that the stronger the smell of the fish, the more fatty acids they contain.
- Poultry like chicken and turkey are the common protein sources.
- Minimal lean red meat with excess fat cut off.
- Dairy products like yogurt, Greek yogurt, and a variety of cheeses are a major part.
- Olive oil is a healthy fat and replaces the more unhealthy, over processed oils like vegetable or canola oil.

The Mediterranean diet does not follow one single plan. In general, it boasts healthy fats, plant proteins, low sugar, and reduced saturated fats as a whole. Along with the food groups mentioned above, the diet also makes sure to utilize a variety of herbs and spices like black pepper, red chili pepper, garlic, ginger, oregano, cumin, coriander, cilantro, parsley, and basil. These extra ingredients add major flavor to the foods which eliminate the need for things like excess salt and grease. Those of you who are carnivores and will miss not having your major portions of meat, with so many flavorful ingredients, most people do not miss the extra meat.

When you eat a hamburger, french fries, pizza, or other greasy food, it tastes good, but the aftereffects will creep up on you, and we are not just speaking of the health consequences. We are mentioning how these foods will make you feel. Generally, you will feel bloated, sluggish, heavy, and maybe even sick hours later. Food is not supposed to make you feel worse. However, many people will devour large amounts of unhealthy foods before they realize what it will do to them. With the Mediterranean diet, you will not have to worry about this. The healthy ingredients involved in the creation of these dishes will make you feel full, but not wear you out.

We will get into the specifics of these recipes later on. There will be many you can choose from. For now, we wanted to discuss some common foods that you can start incorporating into your everyday meal plan.

But for now, some common cuisines considered whole meals are:

- Falafel (a fried patty made from chickpeas)
- Chicken kabob
- Greek salad
- Lamb kabob
- Shakshuka
- Assorted stews
- Numerous types of smoothies, juices and yogurt drinks

Foods To Avoid

There is a wide variety of food groups and ingredients in the Mediterranean diet. You will never have a shortage of what you can eat. That being said there are also many types of food that we must avoid. These foods contain excess sugar, salt and unhealthy saturated fats. Here is a summary of foods that should be avoided:

- Heavily processed foods including meats, as they contain excess salt and other preservatives that are not beneficial for you.
- Butter and margarine
- Refined grains like white bread and white rice do not contain nearly the same nutritional value as whole grains.
- Anything with added sugar like sodas, canned juices, cakes, ice cream, and table sugar.
- Refined oils like canola oil and vegetable oil should be avoided and replaced with healthier options.

If you are to use canned fruit and vegetables, it is recommended that you rinse them thoroughly after opening. Of course, fresh ingredients should always be a priority one. You will notice once you begin tasting Mediterranean cuisine and how it makes you feel, you will stop craving unhealthier options.

Olive Oil Power

The cooking oil you will repeatedly see listed in this book and most common with Mediterranean cooking is olive oil. Namely, extra virgin olive oil, which is the least processed and refined. There is a reason olive oil is popular in the healthiest diet in the world as it has great powers and benefits. Since you will be using this in almost every recipe, let's discuss it more now. The following are some of the benefits to olive oil:

1. Extracted from olives, oleic acid is the primary fatty acid, and many studies suggest it is powerful in reducing inflammation.
2. Olive oil contains large amounts of antioxidants. Antioxidants help reduce the risk of chronic disease.

They also fight inflammation and help with cholesterol, which are two benefits that may lower the risk of heart disease.

3. Olive oil may prevent strokes. Several studies demonstrate that people who consume olive oil on a regular basis are less at risk.
4. Olive oil can help with excess clotting and improves the lining of blood vessels. It has also been shown to lower blood pressure. All of these play a factor in preventing heart disease.
5. Unlike other oils, there seems to be no known link between olive oil and obesity.
6. It may help with the effects of Alzheimer's. There is not a lot of research available yet to support this claim, but the evidence is there.
7. Olive can reduce type 2 diabetes. Several studies have shown that it increases blood sugar and insulin sensitivity.
8. Many antioxidants in olive oil have anti-cancer properties. These antioxidants can reduce oxidative damage due to free radicals, which is believed to be a leading driver of cancer.
9. Olive oil can help treat rheumatoid arthritis because of its strong anti-inflammatory qualities.
10. This type of oil also has antibacterial properties. The nutrients here can inhibit or kill harmful bacteria.

As a side note, another major liquid fat utilized in the Mediterranean diet is avocado oil. This oil has many of the same properties as olive oil and some people prefer the taste of it over other fats. Both of these healthy fats can be incorporated in your diet plan and you cannot go wrong with either one.

Superfoods

A common expression you will hear with healthy diets, including the Mediterranean diet, is the term superfoods. These foods are considered the healthiest of the healthy and are believed to have the capacity to positively affect health.

After learning more from these pages, it won't come as a shock that they are part of the Mediterranean diet, and of course, they would fit into just about anyone's diet plan. Healthy superfoods are the following:

- Kale: Very low in calories, powerful antioxidant and anti-inflammatory properties
- Spinach: Packed with vitamins, has very little taste, and contains anti-cancerous properties
- Blueberries: Tasty and also contains high levels of antioxidants
- Strawberries: More vitamin C than oranges and low in natural sugar
- Greek yogurt: Double the protein of regular yogurt and half the carbs
- Cucumber: Incredible detoxifier for the liver and kidneys as it is 95% water
- Lemon: Healthy and adds some zest
- Bananas: Rich in potassium and fiber and gives a lot of natural energy
- Turmeric: High anti-inflammatory and antioxidant properties
- Ginger: Aids in digestion and supports the immune system
- Chia or flax seeds: Rich in omega-3 fatty acids and fiber
- Avocados: Very nutrient-dense and considered a healthy fat

There are various lists out there of superfoods and you may even find a few more beyond these. The bottom line is, this is a great place to start and consuming a wide variety of these foods will help create optimal health outcomes. Nutrition goes well beyond the confines of the latest dietary trend. Eating healthy should become a regular staple in your life.

Shopping

One of the great things about the Mediterranean diet is that it consists of mainly fresh produce and ingredients from the earth they can be found just about anywhere. You can find them in most grocery stores, specialty and health food stores. Also, online shopping is a common option now and you can have these ingredients shipped to you directly. Unlike many years prior, the ingredients are readily available.

Notes:

Chapter 2: The Healthiest Diet Plan?

There is a common disorder affecting people of all ages, known as chronic inflammation or inflammatory disease. In general, our bodies contain an immune system that works to keep us safe from disease, infection, and injury. When the body senses a foreign substance or some type of injury, it releases various substances such as white blood cells and other chemicals to help fight off a threat. An example of the inflammatory process is when we cut ourselves on something. Immediately, we feel pain, experience redness, and swelling. This is all caused by the chemicals that are released from injured tissues on alert and attract various white blood cells. These white blood cells will attack and subdue any threat that may still exist and then begin the healing process. The engorgement of blood in the area is what also causes warmth and swelling. Whether it is an injury or an infection, our immune systems are working 24/7 to keep us safe from harm.

Acute inflammation is a normal and necessary process to protect our bodies from harm. If these actions did not exist, wounds would be allowed to fester, and infections would spread easier. Not only that, numerous threats to our vital organs and tissues would go unchecked, and our bodies would slowly start getting destroyed. It is amazing just how much our immune systems do to keep us healthy through the inflammatory process. Unfortunately, in this case, too much of a good thing can become a bad thing. In fact, it can even be fatal. When inflammation goes beyond the acute stage, it becomes a chronic issue and can lead to disease. This disease may be a result of normal inflammation lasting too long, or inflammation occurring even without any type of threat. In the event of extended acute inflammation, the body has not gotten rid of whatever caused the acute inflammation. For example, an infection that the body never was able to control. In other cases, the immune system overreacts attacking our cells and tissues, instead of a foreign invader. In instances of inflammatory disease, excessive inflammation causes many long-term issues.

When inflammation occurs without any type of illness or injury, it is because our immune system is misguided, and perceives some type of internal threat that is not there. This is called an autoimmune disorder. Our immune system jumps into action and releases white blood cells and other agents to help protect our bodies. However, since there is no threat, there is nothing for our immune system to fight off. As a result, our own immune system may start attacking our own internal tissues and organs. This will lead to many chronic illnesses in the future, including heart disease, lung disease, digestive issues, kidney failure, skin problems, and neurological disorders.

Consider this example: If your car is parked in a public space with an activated alarm, it is safe, for the most part. If somebody tries to break in, the alarm will sound, you will be alerted and signaled to take care of the intruder. Whether that means scaring them off or calling the authorities. Whatever the case, the intruder is responded to as a threat. This is the same way our immune system works. Something foreign invades our bodies, the immune response is activated, and activates. Now, look at it from another angle. Let's say nothing happens to your car, yet the alarm goes off. We are alerted and react, springing into action. You jump into action, hitting the car thinking there is something wrong but there isn't. But you keep hitting it because nothing is telling you to stop. The car eventually gets damaged or destroyed. This is equivalent to an autoimmune response where our immune system fights viciously even when there is nothing to fight.

In a normal immune response, the attack stops once the threat is neutralized. After this, the rebuilding process begins. When the immune system continues to respond to a nonexistent foreign body without intervention, our internal tissues and organs can be destroyed one by one.

We only witness the results of inflammation superficially in the form of redness, swelling, pain, and heat. However, the same processes occur viscerally to our vital organs. Imagine the damage this can create if it goes untreated. The signs and symptoms of chronic illness can vary and also be quite subtle. They depend on which part of the body is affected. The following are a few signs and symptoms of chronic inflammation or inflammatory disease:

- Fatigue
- Mouth Sores
- Chest Pain
- Difficulty breathing
- Abdominal pain
- Fever
- Rash and dryness
- Joint pain
- Memory problems

The best way to describe inflammation is not so much a disease, but the response to a disease, injury or illness. If left unchecked or uncontrolled will lead to more serious illness. Essentially, inflammation that is left unchecked will lead to widespread swelling and dysfunction throughout the body due to every tissue and vital area of the body being attacked. Some of the diseases that result from chronic inflammation include:

- Asthma
- Stomach ulcers
- Rheumatoid arthritis
- Periodontitis

- Crohn's disease
- Hepatitis
- Coronary artery disease
- Kidney failure
- Stroke
- Heart attack

We are not being hyperbolic when we say that inflammatory disease causes serious health consequences. The results are very real and if we suspect inflammatory disease, we need to nip it in the bud as soon as we can.

There are many ways we can slow down and even prevent chronic inflammation. These include exercise, reducing stress, and getting enough sleep. In more serious cases, medical interventions may be necessary. One of the easiest and most effective methods is changing our dietary habits. You may have been wondering why we went so in-depth into inflammation. We hope we did not put you to sleep because there is a method to our madness. Showcasing the effects of poor health highlights just how valuable a proper diet plan is.

The anti-inflammatory diet is a major defender against the effects of inflammatory disease. This meal plan is marked by several healthy food groups and ingredients that have many anti-inflammatory properties. They will work to prevent inflammatory disease and ultimately reduce the risk of many chronic illnesses.

Why the Mediterranean Diet?

The Mediterranean diet is considered the Mecca of anti-inflammatory diet plans. This is because many of the ingredients are extremely healthy and have strong anti-inflammatory properties. The various food groups, as well as the herbs and spices, have anti-inflammatory properties. Eating the Mediterranean diet regularly will help to prevent many chronic illnesses and pump up energy levels each day. As mentioned before, the healthy ingredients in this diet will fill you up, unlike much of the greasy and heavy food people eat normally. The Mediterranean diet will not make you think you need a nap, instead, you will feel like you have the strength to keep going all day.

Imagine for a moment: You are starving by lunchtime, but you have a lot much more work to get done, but if you don't eat something you feel you will pass out. The only issue is, your normal meal at this time makes you even more tired. But when eating from this diet, you actually feel better. You get a burst of energy and accomplish more than you first planned. A healthy diet plan can certainly help you achieve this vision. If that is not motivation enough, then think about the health benefits.

Imagine not having a heart attack at a young age because you were able to lower your cholesterol, improve your blood pressure, drop a significant amount of weight by an increase in activity. You wake up, move around, and don't have to deal with the same chronic pain issues that were debilitating in the past. This would significantly increase your quality of life. Finally, imagine not feeling bloated, and having improved digestion. People do not give their digestive health enough credit, but it is a major contributor to your overall wellbeing. Eating from the Mediterranean diet regularly can create these outcomes for you. You may even begin seeing results within a couple of days. If this does not inspire you into transitioning to this super diet, I don't know what will.

Let's be real here, health requires some time, effort and money. There is something more expensive and time-consuming than good health, and that is poor health. Hospital stays, medications, missed work days add up over time. Getting that one-dollar cheeseburger at the drive-thru may seem economical in the moment, but after some time, it won't seem that financially smart. The next time you find yourself complaining about the cost of healthy food, consider for a moment, the ultimate cost of unhealthy food.

We are certainly not saying you cannot indulge once in a while. All of us love our certain "bad" foods. We encourage cheat meals and cheat days. Just don't let it get out of hand. Cheat days can turn into cheat weeks, cheat months, and cheat years. We need to be careful and practice some discipline.

History

The Mediterranean diet has been around for thousands of years and originates from the various countries that surround the region outside of the Mediterranean Sea. Many researchers have traced the diet going back to the years of AD, well before the common era, where several Greek physicians who followed the studies of Hippocrates attributed various foods to promoting good health. Hippocrates, who is considered the father of modern medicine, is one of the first known physicians who did not attribute illness and disease to unknown paranormal or supernatural forces. His medical practices were based on observing the human body and its functions. His core belief in medicine was that illnesses had a physical component that could be explained rationally. Prior to Hippocrates, many people, including physicians, assumed that illnesses were a punishment from the Gods and could not be rectified. The beliefs of Hippocrates began to change this mindset.

Several centuries after Hippocrates, a Greek physician named Aelius Galenus, or simply, Galen, was a major proponent of preventative medicine and saw diet and nutrition as equal to pharmacology in the way they prevent diseases. Galen also believed that the more flavorful the food, the better the nutritional content. He would often instruct his patients to season their food with various herbs and spices like pepper and ginger. While many of the ingredients utilized in the Mediterranean diet today were not readily available in Galen's time, much of the foundation of the cuisine was laid by these Greek physicians that are still applied over 2,000 years later. For example, Galen and other hippocratic physicians discouraged high fat and sugar intake on a regular basis. It is safe to say that the structural groundwork was formed by Galen for what would become one of the healthiest diets in history.

The health benefits of the diet started coming into prominence in the 1960s when Ancel Keys, Ph.D., from the University of Minnesota began extensive research on the health outcomes of 13,000 men throughout various countries in the world. Through this research, it was found that men from the Mediterranean region had much lower rates of cardiovascular disease than their counterparts in other countries, including Japan, Northern Europe, and the United States. This caught the attention of many individuals in the medicine and scientific world. Ever since then, this diverse meal plan has gained much more interest throughout the world.

Continued research is being conducted to learn the extensive benefits this diet holds. Scientists are finding more evidence that the Mediterranean diet has an array of health benefits, including increased life span, healthy weight loss, improved memory, lower risks of certain cancers and diabetes, decreased blood pressure, and lower cholesterol levels. Hundreds of studies have been done showcasing these results since the original one with Dr. Keys. The science is still out in many ways, however, the evidence thus far is certainly lopsided towards it being a healthy diet plan. Today, the Mediterranean diet has grown and it is difficult to go to any country, especially those with major metropolitan areas, and not find some form of Mediterranean cuisine available. This diet boasts simple, plant-based food that is nutrient-dense and comes from a localized area. The more that this diet gets incorporated into people's routines, the better the outcome. Of course, this is considering people stick to the traditional diet with authentic ingredients.

With the passing of time so have risen the countless diet plans that seem to pop up every week. Some of them are legitimate for their own reasons, and others are just fads or crash diets offering no long-term benefits. The Mediterranean diet is the one meal plan that consistently offers high-quality foods and dietary plans with improved outcomes. Since the Mediterranean diet has been around a while, it is also the most well-researched. The following are a few diet plans that are often compared to our super diet. While there are some similarities, there are significant differences too.

- Flexitarian Diet: Also known as the flexible vegetarian diet. This diet promotes vegetables, whole grains, and healthy oils. While animal products are allowed, they are not encouraged as much as plant-based proteins. This diet is quite similar to the Mediterranean diet.
- Keto Diet: Many people compare this diet to the Mediterranean diet because of the high fat intake. However, this is much more fat content in the keto diet. In addition, many different carbohydrates like whole grains, legumes, and fruits are off-limits. The keto diet is also not very sustainable because it is much more restrictive than the Mediterranean and flexitarian diets.
- The DASH Diet: The acronym stands for Dietary Approaches to Stop Hypertension. This diet is also

quite similar to the Mediterranean diet as it promotes a lot of whole grains, lean meats, fruits, and vegetables. The main difference is that this diet puts more emphasis on low-fat dairy and proteins.

Our super diet closely resembles the USDA dietary guidelines. The major differences are the higher promotion of whole grains, and the use of non-animal proteins. The USDA states that half of your grains should be whole, while the Mediterranean diet encourages whole grains. Furthermore, the USDA treats all proteins the same, while this gives less value to red meats.

At the current stage, the Mediterranean diet is still considered the healthiest meal plan. It boasts all-around healthy ingredients, nutrient-dense food groups, and proper serving sizes. Of course, serving sizes are not as strict, as we will explain further in this book.

Story Time

We feel that some good stories will help us understand just how impeccable this diet plan is. These stories are hypothetical scenarios, however, based on the benefits, these tales showcase just how Mediterranean cuisine can be life-changing. Yes, life-changing. Visualise this:

Johnny

Johnny is a high-level CEO at a major firm, and only 30 years old. He makes a good living and enjoys the perks of travel and eating in the finest restaurants. He owns a beautiful home in the suburbs and can afford to do basically anything. From the outside looking in, it seems like Johnny has a perfect life. However, it is really impossible to have it all. At some point, you have to give something up. For him, this was his health.

Due to his busy schedule, Johnny didn't pay much attention to what he was eating, or his activity levels. His meals consisted of fast food, sugary drinks, and a lot of bread, pasta, or pizza. This food sustained him, but his energy levels would crash mid day. To pick himself up, he would drink energy drinks. Johnny never felt the effects of this lifestyle as a young man. At least, not on the outside.

Over the past year, Johnny began waking up with headaches, and his joints, back, and neck became stiff and hurt throughout the day. This was beginning to hurt his workflow and activities of daily living. No matter how much or how well he slept, he would still wake up feeling sluggish and in pain. His pain was getting worse by the day. He was also gaining quite a bit of weight. He was close to about 20 pounds more than the previous year.

After a while, Johnny began having difficulty breathing, exerting himself, and his pain continued to grow. One of his friends, who was quite concerned about him, recommended eating better foods. She began introducing him to the Mediterranean diet, which he resisted at first. Johnny was used to eating his "feel good" food. He was not ready to give them up, even though what he was actually feeling was miserable. He was not convinced that the new diet his friend was offering would help. Eventually, she convinced Johnny to try a few different foods, and he was thoroughly impressed.

She encouraged him to stick to it for a couple of days and see how he felt. And after the second day, much to Johnny's surprise, he felt less sluggish and his joints were hurting a little less. He still craved his old foods, so Johnny's friend decided to help put him on a plan to transition to the

Mediterranean diet. She had made the change a few months earlier and was feeling better than ever before.

She began helping Johnny by having him change one meal every day to something that followed the diet guidelines. This was either a main meal or a snack. Sometimes, it was just one type of food in a meal. After two weeks, Johnny fully transitioned to the Mediterranean diet. He already had more energy, less pain in his joints, was sleeping better, and no longer woke up with headaches. After two more solid weeks eating the super diet, Johnny was down 15 pounds, felt much more energized, barely had any pain in his joints, and was walking and moving around with no issues. His productivity at work was back up too.

After experiencing this dramatic shift, Johnny swore his past diet completely. He was not fully engaged with the Mediterranean meal plan. The food was delicious and the amazing way he felt was worth not going back to his old ways. He even had more energy to do activities after work, which he did not even have when he was younger. Johnny's story is a major example of how the Mediterranean diet can improve your quality of life. The food groups can truly work miracles if you allow them to.

Susan

Susan worked as a nurse at a local hospital. She enjoyed taking care of patients but would be deeply affected when any passed away. The majority of these patients were much older than her, so she would not think about their health complications. Due to her busy schedule, Susan rarely took the time to eat, or drink water. For energy she would eat something quick like a candy bar or a sip of an instant cappuccino. Susan was always tired, and her back was always aching. She would regularly experience muscle pain impeding her mobility. And the problems were getting worse.

One day, a coworker warned her that her pain could be the result of something internal. She figured it was just because she needed to rest. However, even when she got enough sleep and took several days off, she was still in a lot of pain, feeling sluggish, and regularly experiencing headaches. She also began having chest pain that put her in the ER. The workup at the hospital concluded it was stress-related.

Because of this, Susan went on with her current lifestyle and bad eating habits. She had no intention of changing anything, despite her doctors and coworker's warnings. One afternoon, a patient arrived on their floor who was quite young, a couple of years younger than Susan. She was obese with many corresponding health complications. Susan got to know this patient well and even took a liking to her. After a couple of days, the patient ended up passing away due to heart disease. Susan was distraught over this.

A few days later, Susan had an epiphany. She realized that could have been her. She could be the one who died on the hospital bed due to poor health. The ER visit from before was a warning sign she did not recognize. After this, Susan promised herself she would make some changes. With the help of her coworker, she learned about healthy diet plans and came upon the Mediterranean diet.

Slowly, Susan began incorporating food from the diet into her meals. Just one or two meals a day for several days made a big difference. She already noticed that she had more natural energy than before. After about a month, she was eating meals from the Mediterranean diet throughout the day and she would also find time to sit down and eat, which was major for her. After the first month, Susan had no more aches or pains, including no more chest pain. She felt like a whole new person after transitioning into this diet plan.

With the increased energy, Susan was even able to start exercising regularly. She was on her way to potentially fatal health problems, but luckily after she changed her diet, she avoided catastrophe. Susan's story shows that the Mediterranean diet can help prevent many chronic illnesses.

Phil

Phil was a hard worker and also very careful with his money. He barely ever spent a dime, especially on himself. He hated wasting money. Phil usually ate fast food because it was quick, easy and barely affected his wallet. The various value menus would provide him meals for days on end. He had no interest in spending several dollars on a salad when he could get a burger for less than half the price and feel full.

Phil knew this was bad for his health, but he was not interested in spending the time and money it took for a proper diet. He didn't think it was worth the price. For years, Phil thought he was doing the right thing. If you looked at it superficially, he certainly was saving himself thousands of dollars on wasted food.

One morning, Phil was not feeling well. He ached all over, in his bones and muscles, and was having chest pain. He ended up going to the emergency room. While there, the staff ran tests to determine the cause. Upon completion, they found that his labs were quite abnormal, his inflammation biomarkers were elevated, and his scans showed some concerning sights. The bottom line is, he had prediabetes, high blood pressure, slight swelling of the outer lining of the heart, known as pericarditis, and even his labs showing kidney function were elevated, showing possible disease in this area. Needless to say, Phil was in bad shape and it's safe to say his diet for so many years played a major part. Phil never received the proper nutrition he sorely needed. He just wanted a quick meal all of the time that was cheap.

As Phil layed in bed wondering what happened. He thought about having to lay in the emergency room, how much time he would be spending at various doctor's offices from now on, and how much money he would be spending on medications to keep himself alive and healthy. Furthermore, he would have to stop eating fast food and actually begin going for healthier options. He realized at this moment, that his unhealthy dietary choices actually cost him more money in the long run. He would be paying the price for it for the rest of his life.

Many people are so concerned about what a healthy lifestyle will cost them. It is the most unusual element to put a price tag on. This is not a book about finance, however, if you are going to go cheap on something, pick something different than your own well-being.

James

James was overweight. He had been this way since he was a kid and it seemed there was nothing, he could do about it. No matter how active he was, he never was able to lose weight. This annoyed him to the core, but he was used to it. He went on various different diet plans, exercise programs, and avoided stress and anything unhealthy as best as he could. Unfortunately, it did not make a difference and he actually ended up gaining.

He tried every different fad diet that would come out but none of them worked. If they did, it was very short-lived. James exercised constantly, but it also did nothing to help him. Whatever combination of exercise and diet he pursued, the results were always the same, stagnation. One of the issues was that James would not last on certain diets because he would have to deprive himself of so much.

James' health continued to get worse as he gained weight seemingly every week. He was suffering from painful joints, and when he went to the doctor, he was discovered to have mild hypertension. James was ready to give up, because nothing he did made any difference. It was a broken record.

One day, one of James' friends, who was a dietician, filled him in on the Mediterranean diet plan. James never heard that phrase, but when he began reading about the ingredients, he knew he had heard of it before. He may have even tried some variation of it. His friend went over the diet in detail and all of the ingredients, food groups and meals that would be involved. James liked what he was hearing. The food sounded good, even though he did not know what most of it was.

James and his friend set up a meal plan that would have him slowly incorporate aspects of the diet into his routine. After the first week, about half of his meals followed the appropriate diet plan. By about the third week, he was fully engaged in the Mediterranean diet. The food was delicious, and he enjoyed the diversity of flavors. The best part was how it made him feel. James began having more energy than he had in decades. His pain symptoms were going away, and he was even losing weight. He could not believe this. This was the first time in his life that he noticeably lost weight and felt slimmer. Switching to the Mediterranean diet full time is just what he needed to do.

The main reason the diet worked so well for James is because he was not depriving himself of anything. He was able to get all of the nutrients he needed with the diversity of the meal plans. Everyday for every meal, James was able to eat something new. He even began making his own meals, including a daily smoothie. After several months, James is continuing on the dietary plan and not looking back.

Do you find yourself in similar situations that we illustrated in the stories above. It may not be too late to change your path. Get the proper medical advice and begin incorporating the Mediterranean diet and lifestyle into your daily routine. You may start feeling better within a couple of days.

The Mediterranean Diet and Medical Diets

When patients are admitted into the hospital, they are often put on various diets based on their particular health concerns. One of these diets is the cardiac diet, which promotes low salt, low cholesterol, low sugar, and low fat. The purpose is to prevent further damage to the heart and its supporting organs. The cardiac diet, actually resembles the Mediterranean diet, however, it does not promote the same nutrient density and variety of foods available. In addition, the flavors are not nearly as bold. If the mediterranean diet could be further incorporated into the medical system, the health outcomes may even be better.

There is another major diet plan out there, and it is known as the renal diet, or kidney diet. It also contains many of the same restrictions as the cardiac diet, and further restricts excess fluid, potassium, phosphorus, and various other nutrients. The reason is because the kidneys cannot filter them out like before and a heavy build-up of these substances can lead to major health concerns and even death. So, there are numerous restrictions with the renal diet.

The same holds true for the diabetic diet and so many other medically necessary diets. The interesting thing is, these diets are based on restrictions, while the Mediterranean diet promotes an abundance of food. There are certainly food groups that are not recommended, however, there is rarely any restriction on nutrients.

This is one of the main reasons the Mediterranean diet is so sustainable. When people switch, they won't miss anything. Our bodies are quite interesting in the sense that they know what they need. When we learn to listen to our bodies carefully, we can understand what is missing and what is in abundance. For example, feelings of bloatedness and sluggishness may indicate having too much fat and cholesterol in our diets, while missing out on many other ingredients. With the Mediterranean diet, you will stop feeling your body in discomfort, because it will give the body what it needs.

Notes:

Chapter 3: The Mediterranean Diet Recipes

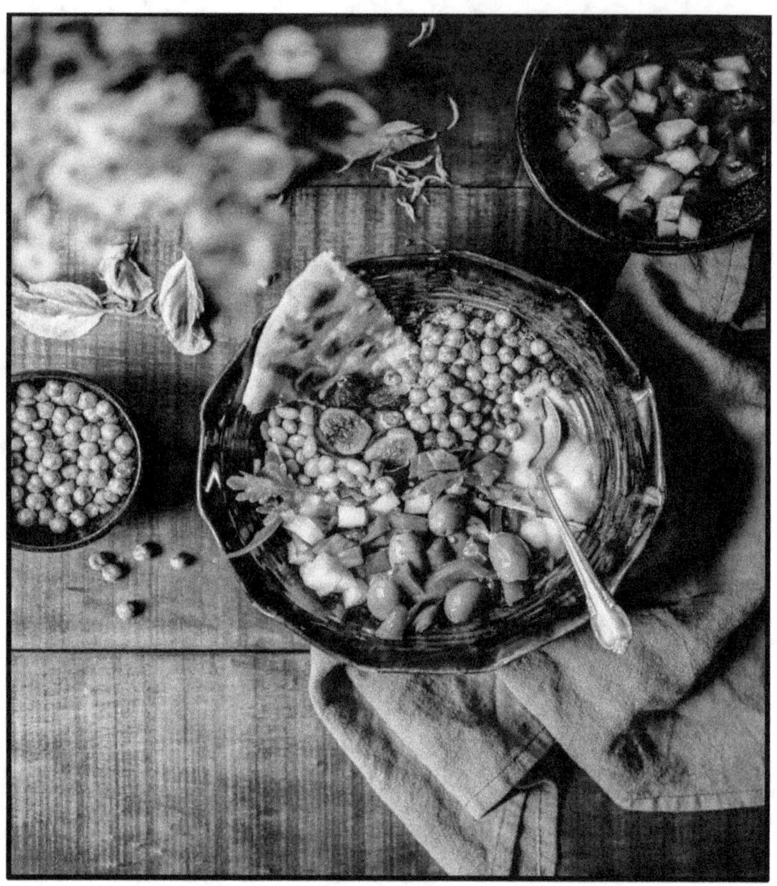

We have discussed the Mediterranean diet extensively. We have detailed what it is, where it comes from, and the many health benefits that it has. We will now provide you with a number of delicious recipes that you can try for yourself. We will provide all of the necessary ingredients you will need, plus step by step instructions on how to prepare the delicious food. We will break this down into separate sections to showcase different varieties of meal plans.

Before we begin giving you recipes, we wanted to list some of the most common ingredients found in the Mediterranean diet for you to keep an eye out for.

- Broccoli Rabe
- Chickpeas
- Eggplant
- Olive oil
- Cumin powder
- Coriander powder
- Black pepper
- Red pepper
- Paprika
- bell peppers
- Tomato
- Seafood
- Chicken
- Wheat
- Olives
- Capers
- Lemons
- Lean red meats
- Ginger
- Garlic

Of course, there are other ingredients, these are just some of the key ingredients used in most meal plans. Use these ingredients to your liking to create tasty and healthy cuisines that will fill you up each time. The recipes below are just examples of how you can mix these ingredients together to make magic. Cooking is an art form, just like painting, so get creative with these recipes and feel free to make your own. With our recipes, we will mainly be using olive oil. However, as we mentioned before, avocado oil can be an acceptable replacement in many situations.

Main Dishes

In this first section, we will provide the recipe for several main dishes. These are typically for lunch or dinner. There is a separate section for breakfast.

Eggplant, Lentils, Peppers in Olive Oil

Total Time: 75 Minutes

Servings: 4

Nutrition Facts:

Calories-197 kcal

Total Fats-8 g

Protein-7 g

Carbohydrates: 29 g

Ingredients:

- 6 oz rinsed green lentils
- 2 medium eggplants
- 4 cloves of garlic
- 1 red bell pepper, cut in half
- 14 oz can of diced tomatoes
- 4 tbsp extra virgin olive oil
- 1 cup of water
- 3 more Tbsp extra virgin olive oil
- 1 tsp salt
- 1 tsp granulated sugar
- 4 tsp dried mint
- Freshly ground black pepper to taste

Instructions:

1. Put the green lentils in a pan of boiling water, stir, and cover. Simmer on low heat for 15 minutes, drain the water and set aside.
2. With a peeler, peel the eggplants in zebra stripes. Cut the eggplant in half lengthwise and then cut each half into medium slices. Spread them out over a wide tray, sprinkle your salt over them and leave aside for 15 minutes. Using a paper towel, gently squeeze the excess water out of the eggplants.
3. In a pan, add 3 tbsp olive oil and heat on medium, then lightly sauté the prepared eggplant for 1-2 minutes.
4. In a large bowl, combine the lentils from before, onion, garlic, bell peppers, tomatoes. salt, dried mint, the remaining olive oil, and sugar. Season with ground black pepper to taste.
5. In a wide, heavy pan, place a layer of the eggplant slices. Spread half of the vegetable mixture over the eggplant evenly. Place the remaining eggplant over the top of this mixture and then spread the remaining mixture over this. Add the water, cover and cook on low to medium heat for 35 minutes.
6. Once cooked, cover and cool the dish in the pan. This will allow the flavors to develop.
7. Serve at room temperature.

Ratatouille

Total Time: 85 minutes

Servings: 10

Nutrition Facts:

Calories: 80 kcal

Total Fats: 3.4 g

Proteins: 2.5 g

Carbohydrates: 11.9 g

Ingredients:

- 2 tbsp extra virgin olive oil
- 2 coarsely chopped onions
- 2 bell peppers, red or yellow
- 4 minced garlic cloves
- 1 ½ tsp crushed fennel seeds
- 1 medium diced eggplant
- 2 large diced zucchinis
- 6 chopped tomatoes
- ¼ cup finely chopped fresh basil
- 2 tbsp finely chopped fresh thyme
- Salt to taste
- Freshly ground black pepper to taste

Instructions:

1. Turn on the oven ahead of time and preheat to 350 degrees-F.
2. Add one tbsp olive oil to a pot and cook over medium heat. Add bell peppers and onions and cook, while stirring occasionally, for 8-10 minutes. Add garlic and fennel seeds, and cook for another 1 minute. Transfer these vegetables to a large bowl.
3. Add ½ tbsp olive oil and then add the eggplant. Cook about 7-8 minutes until lightly browned and then transfer to a bowl with other vegetables.
4. Add the remaining olive oil to the pot. Add zucchini and cook, stirring frequently until lightly browned. Add tomatoes, basil, thyme, and cooked vegetables from before. Bring to a simmer, cover the pot and transfer to the preheated oven.
5. Bake the ratatouille, stirring occasionally until the vegetables are tender. This usually takes 35-45 minutes.
6. Sprinkle salt and pepper for flavoring to taste. You may garnish with parsley if desired. Serve hot or at room temperature.

Oven Roasted Chicken Shawarma

Total Time: 70 minutes

Servings: 8

Nutrition Facts:

Calories: 214 kcal

Total Fats: 17 g

Proteins: 10 g

Carbohydrates: 4 g

Ingredients:

Chicken Shawarma

- 4 tbsp freshly squeezed lemon juice
- ½ cup olive oil
- 1 tsp salt
- 2 tsp ground cumin
- 2 tsp ground black pepper
- 2 tsp smoked paprika
- ½ tsp turmeric
- 1 tsp red pepper flakes
- ½ tsp cinnamon
- 4 cloves of minced garlic
- 3 boneless and skinless chicken breasts
- 1 large sliced onion
- 2 tbsp fresh parsley for garnish

Garlic Sauce

- 1 cup of vegetable oil
- ⅓ cup lemon juice
- 6 cloves of peeled garlic
- 1 egg white
- 1 tsp salt

Instructions:

Chicken Shawarma

1. In a large bowl, add garlic, lemon juice, olive oil, salt, cumin, turmeric, red pepper flakes, black pepper, paprika, and cinnamon. Whisk all ingredients well.
2. Make sure the chicken is well-coated by adding it to the marinade mixture and tossing it well. Refrigerate for minimum one hour after covering it with foil.
3. Preheat the oven to 425 degrees-F. Remove the bowl with chicken and marinade from the refrigerator, add sliced onion and toss well so that the onion is fully coated. Spread the contents of the bowl evenly on a 9x13 baking dish.
4. Bake until the chicken is brown and crispy on the edges, which will take 40-45 minutes.
5. Let the chicken cool down for 5 minutes and then shred into small bits.

Garlic Sauce

1. Add ingredients for garlic sauce to a high-quality blender and process 1-2 minutes, or until smooth.
2. Serve with chicken as desired.

Baked Lemon Garlic Cod

Total Time: 19 minutes

Servings: 4

Nutrition Facts:

Calories: 258 kcal

Total Fats: 6 g

Proteins: 38 g

Carbohydrates: 12 g

Ingredients:

- 4-6 oz boneless and skinless pieces of cod
- Sea salt to taste
- Freshly ground black pepper to taste
- 1 ½ tsp butter
- 1 tbsp olive oil
- 2 crushed garlic cloves
- 2 tbsp lemon juice
- 2 tbsp parsley chopped

Ingredients:

1. Preheat the oven to 400 degrees-F.
2. Place cod pieces in a baking dish large enough to fit all 4 in one layer. Lightly coat the bottom of the dish with cooking spray.
3. Season fish with sea salt and black pepper to taste.
4. Place butter and garlic oil in a small non-stick skillet. Heat on medium and add garlic. Sauté for 1 minute. Add lemon juice and parsley and remove from heat.
5. Drizzle garlic mixture over top of cod pieces.
6. Bake for 12-14 minutes. Cod should flake easily using a fork. Ready to serve!

Seafood Paella

Total Time: 65 minutes

Servings: 6

Nutrition Facts:

Calories: 357.2

Total fats: 10.1 g

Proteins: 19.2 g

Carbohydrates: 46.2 g

Ingredients:

- 4 ½ cups of chicken stock
- ½ tsp saffron threads, crumbled
- ¼ tsp salt
- 3 tbsp olive oil
- ½ finely chopped yellow onion
- ½ finely chopped red bell pepper
- 3 cloves finely chopped garlic
- 6 oz mild dried chorizo sausage, sliced into thin half-moons
- 3 cups short-grained rice
- 14 oz can of fire-roasted diced tomatoes
- 1 cup frozen peas
- 1 pound of large shrimp, peeled and deveined with tail left on
- 1 pound mussels, rinsed and scrubbed
- 1 pound littleneck clams, rinsed and scrubbed
- ¼ cup of chopped parsley for garnish

Instructions:

1. Heat up a gas grill to 375 degrees-F.
2. Bring the stock to a boil using medium heat in a saucepan. Add saffron and salt. After turning off the heat, let the saffron steep for 15 minutes.
3. Add oil to a 14-inch steel skillet, and turn the stove to medium heat. Add the red pepper and onions, cook 5-7 minutes until onions are translucent. Stir in garlic and chorizo.
4. Add the sofrito, rice, tomatoes, infused stock, salt, peas, shrimp, mussels, and clams to a skillet.
5. Set the skillet with sofrito on the grill, add rice, and cook, stirring often for 4-5 minutes. Stir in the stock, tomatoes, and peas. Taste and add more salt if needed. Spread the rice evenly over the bottom of the pan. close the grill and simmer the rice for 15 minutes. Do not stir yet.
6. With the hinge sides up, nestle the clams and mussels into the rice. This will allow the juices to be

released into the rice. Arrange so the shrimp is around the shellfish.

7. Cover the pan with foil, close the grill and cook for 6-10 minutes, or until the rice and shrimp are cooked through and the mussels and clams are open.
8. Use a spatula to pick up rice and see if you have achieved the brown crispy bottom or socarrat. If not, cook uncovered for a few more minutes to lightly caramelize the bottom.
9. Sprinkle with parsley and it is ready to serve.

Spanakopita (Greek Spinach Pie)

Total Time: 80 minutes

Servings: 12

Nutrition Facts:

Calories: 393 kcal

Total Fats: 20.6 g

Proteins: 21.4 g

Carbohydrates: 38.8 g

Ingredients:

Filling

- 16 oz frozen chopped spinach, thawed and well-drained
- 2 bunches of flat-leaf parsley, finely chopped
- 1 large finely chopped yellow onion
- 2 minced garlic cloves
- 2 tbsp extra virgin olive oil
- 2 tsp dry dill weed
- 4 eggs
- 10.5 oz crumbled feta cheese

- Freshly ground black pepper

Crust

- 16 oz package of organic dough, thawed
- 1 cup of extra virgin olive oil

Instructions:

1. Turn the oven to 325 degrees-F to preheat.
2. In a bowl, add the spinach along with all of the other filling ingredients. Stir until well-combined.
3. Unroll the dough sheets and place them between two damp kitchen cloths.
4. Prepare a 9.5x13 inch baking sheet. Brush the bottom and sides with olive oil.
5. Line the inside of the baking dish, including the sides, with the dough. Brush with olive oil and add two more sheets in the same manner. Brush them with olive oil also. Repeat these steps until ⅔ of the dough is used up.
6. Evenly spread the prepared filling over the crust. Top with two more sheets of dough and brush with olive oil. Continue to layer the sheets and brush with olive oil until all the dough is used up. Over the top layer, lightly brush with olive oil and sprinkle a few drops of water.
7. Fold the excess dough flats from the sides, brush them with olive oil. Cut the spanakopita only part way through into squares. You can also do all of the cutting later, this just adds to the evenness of the cooking.
8. Bake in the preheated oven for 1 hour or until the crust is golden brown. Remove from the oven and finish cutting through the pie dish and serve.

Moroccan Vegetable Tagine

Total Time: 55 minutes

Servings: 4-6

Nutrition Facts:

Calories: 448 kcal

Total fats: 18.4 g

Proteins: 16.9 g

Carbohydrates: 60.7 g

Ingredients:

- ¼ cup extra virgin olive oil
- 2 medium chopped yellow onions
- 8-10 chopped garlic cloves
- 2 large chopped carrots
- 2 large peeled and cubed russet potatoes
- 1 tbsp Harissa spice blend
- 1 tsp ground coriander
- 1 tsp ground cinnamon
- ½ tsp ground turmeric
- 2 cups of canned whole peeled tomatoes
- ½ cup chopped dried apricot
- 1 quart vegetable broth
- 2 cups cooked chickpeas
- Juice from 1 lemon
- A handful of fresh parsley leaves

Instructions:

1. Warm up olive oil in a large pot over medium heat, until oil is shimmering. Add onions and increase to high heat. Sauté for 5 minutes.
2. Add garlic and chopped vegetables. Season with salt and spices. Toss to combine.
3. Mix regularly as you cook for 5-7 minutes on medium to high heat.
4. Add tomatoes, apricot, broth and a dash of salt.

5. Cook for 10 minutes and then reduce heat. Place cover and let simmer for 20-25 minutes. The vegetables should be tender. Carefully add in the chickpeas and cook another 5 minutes on low heat.
6. Stir in lemon juice and fresh parsley. Taste and add more seasoning if needed.
7. Transfer to serving bowls and top each with a drizzle of extra virgin olive oil.

Baked Salmon

Total Time: 15 minutes

Servings: 4

Nutrition Facts:

Calories: 411 kcal

Total Fats: 29.1 g

Proteins: 38.5 g

Carbohydrates: 1.5 g

Ingredients:

- 1 ½ pound fresh Atlantic salmon
- Kosher salt to taste
- Freshly ground black pepper to taste
- 1 cup of fresh cilantro leaves
- 1 cup fresh parsley leaves
- 2 green onions, the tops only
- 1 garlic clove
- ½ cup extra virgin olive oil
- 1 tbsp red wine vinegar
- 1 tbsp fresh lemon juice
- ½ tsp oregano
- ¼ tsp kosher salt for chimichurri sauce

Instructions:

1. Preheat the oven to 450 degrees-F.
2. Sprinkle the salmon with kosher salt and black pepper generously. Place it on a parchment-lined baking sheet.
3. Bake the salmon for about 10 minutes until flaky. Cooking times can vary based on oven variation and thickness of the salmon.
4. To make the chimichurri sauce: Slice off the tops of the green onions. In a blender, add the green onion tops, cilantro, parsley, garlic, olive oil, red wine vinegar, lemon juice, oregano, kosher salt, and black pepper. Blend all ingredients until smooth.
5. Drizzle the chimichurri sauce over the salmon and enjoy.

One-Skillet Mediterranean Chicken

Total Time: 30 minutes

Servings: 5

Nutrition Facts:

Calories: 384 kcal

Total Fats: 26 g

Proteins: 27 g

Carbohydrates: 9 g

Ingredients:

- 1 tbsp olive oil
- Plus 1 tsp olive oil
- 1-½ pounds boneless skinless chicken tenderloins
- 1 medium chopped red onion
- 1 tsp minced garlic
- 1, 15 oz can petite diced tomatoes
- ½ cup California ripe black olives, sliced
- 1 tbsp fresh oregano
- 1 tbsp fresh basil
- 1 cup halved cherry tomatoes

- Salt to your own taste
- Freshly ground black pepper to your own taste

Instructions:

1. In a large cast-iron skillet, heat 1 tbsp of olive oil on medium heat. Add the chicken and sauté until browned throughout, which will take about 10 minutes. Remove the chicken to a plate.
2. Add 1 tsp of olive oil and onions to the skillet. Sauté onions for about 2 minutes on medium heat. Carefully pour in the garlic and cook for an additional minute. Add the canned tomatoes, olives and spices. Cook for another 6-8 minutes.
3. Add the chicken and halved tomatoes, cook all the way through.
4. Serve over rice or potatoes.

Falafel

Total Time: 50 minutes

Servings: 12 patties

Nutrition Facts:

Calories: 93

Total Fats: 3.8 g

Proteins: 3.9 g

Carbohydrates: 1.4 g

Ingredients:

- 2 cups dried chickpeas
- ½ tsp baking soda
- 1 cup fresh parsley leaves
- ¾ cup fresh cilantro leaves
- ¼ cup fresh dill
- 1 small onion cut in quarters
- 7-8 garlic cloves

- 1 tbsp ground black pepper
- Salt to taste
- 1 tbsp ground cumin
- 1 tbsp ground coriander
- 1 tsp cayenne pepper
- 1 tsp baking powder
- 2 tbsp toasted sesame seeds
- Olive oil for frying

Instructions:

1. Place the dried chickpeas and baking soda in a large bowl filled with water. Soak chickpeas overnight for 16-18 hours. Drain the chickpeas and pat dry.
2. Add the chickpeas, herbs, onions, garlic, and spices to the large bowl of a food processor. Process for 40 minutes at a time until all ingredients are well combined.
3. Transfer this falafel mixture to a container and cover tightly. right before frying, add baking powder and fennel seeds to the mixture and stir with a spoon
4. Scoop handfuls of the falafel mixture and form patties.
5. Fill a medium saucepan 3 inches up with oil. Heat on medium until it simmers softly. Carefully drop the falafel patties into the mixture and fry until lightly brown. This will take about 3-5 minutes.
6. Place the falafel patties in a plate lined with paper towels to help drain the oil.
7. The falafel can be eaten alone or in a salad, pita, or sandwich.

Greek Baked Meatballs

Total Time: 80 minutes

Servings: 16 pieces

Nutrition Facts:

Calories: 64 kcal

Total Fats: 2.7 g

Proteins: 2.2 g

Carbohydrates: 7.5 g

Ingredients:

Meatballs

- 2 slice whole-wheat bread, lightly toasted.
- ¼ cup milk
- 1 ½ pound lean ground beef
- 1 chopped small yellow onion
- 3 minced garlic cloves
- 2 medium eggs
- 1 tsp ground cumin
- ½ tsp ground cinnamon
- ½ tsp dried oregano
- ½ cup chopped fresh parsley
- Extra virgin olive oil for drizzle
- Salt and pepper to taste

Red Sauce

- Extra virgin olive oil
- 1 finely chopped yellow onion
- 2 minced garlic cloves
- ½ cup dry red wine
- 30 oz can of tomato sauce
- 1 bay leaf
- ¾ tsp ground cumin
- ½ tsp cinnamon
- ½ tsp sugar
- Salt and pepper to taste

Instructions:

1. Using a small bowl, place the toasted bread and cover with milk to soak. When the bread is soft, squeeze the liquid out completely and discard milk.

2. Transfer the bread to a large mixing bowl. Add ground beef and the rest of the meatball ingredients. Knead well until all combined. Place in the fridge for now.

3. Preheat the oven to 400 degrees-F.

4. To prepare the sauce: In a large skillet, heat 2 tbsp extra virgin olive oil over medium heat until slightly simmering. Add onions and cook for about 3 minutes. Add garlic and cook another minute, while stirring. Now add red wine and cook to reduce wine by about 1/2, then add tomato sauce, bay leaf, and leftover ingredients for sauce. Once boiling, reduce heat and simmer for 15 minutes.

5. Prepare a baking dish and lightly oil the bottom with extra virgin olive oil.

6. Take the mixture out of the fridge and scoop out about 2 ½ tbsp of meat mixture and form into elongated meatballs. You should have enough mixture for 16 meatballs. Arrange the meatballs in the baking dish and cover with sauce. Remove bay leaf from the sauce.

7. Bake in the preheated oven for 40-45 minutes or until meatballs are well-cooked throughout. It is recommended to use the middle rack in the oven. Assess meatballs during the baking process. If they are getting too dry, may add a small amount of water to the dish.

8. Remove from the oven, drizzle olive oil. Garnish with parsley. Serve over rice.

Greek Lemon Rice

Total Time: 45 minutes

Servings: 6

Nutrition Facts:

Calories: 145 kcal

Total Fats: 6.9 g

Proteins: 3.3 g

Carbohydrates: 18.3 g

Ingredients:

- 2 cups long-grain rice
- Extra virgin olive oil
- 1 medium chopped yellow onion
- 1 minced garlic clove
- ½ cup orzo pasta
- Juice from 2 lemons plus one lemon zest
- 2 cups of low-sodium chicken or vegetable broth
- Pinch of salt
- Large handful of chopped fresh parsley
- 1 tsp dill weed

Instructions:

1. Rinse rice thoroughly and then soak in cold water for 15-20 minutes. Drain well.
2. Heat about 3 tbsp extra virgin olive oil on medium in a large saucepan until it is simmering, but not smoking. Carefully add the onions and cook until luminous, which will take about 3-4 minutes. Add uncooked pasta and garlic. Toss around until the orzo has gained some color. Gently stir in the rice and toss to coat completely.
3. Add the lemon juice and broth. Bring liquid to a light boil, then turn heat to low. Conceal the pan and cook for 20 minutes. Rice should be tender, and all liquid should be soaked up.
4. Remove rice from heat. Leave it covered for 10 minutes.
5. Uncover and stir in lemon zest, dill weed, and parsley. Ready to serve!

Mediterranean Grilled Chicken Breast

Total Time: 35 minutes

Servings: 4

Nutrition Facts:

Calories: 820 kcal

Total Fats: 47 g

Proteins: 71 g

Carbohydrates: 31 g

Ingredients:

- 4 boneless skinless chicken breasts cut in half
- 3 tbsp lemon juice
- 3 tbsp olive oil
- 3 tbsp chopped fresh parsley
- 3 crushed garlic cloves
- 1 tsp paprika
- ½ tsp dried oregano
- ½ tsp salt
- ½ teaspoon ground black pepper

Instructions:

1. Combine lemon juice, 2 tbsp olive oil, parsley, garlic, paprika, and oregano in a large plastic food storage bag.
2. Pierce chicken with a fork several times and sprinkle salt and pepper. Add chicken to bag and coat with dressing. Marinate for 20 minutes.
3. Remove chicken from the bag. Add 1 tbsp olive oil to the grill pan, and place on medium heat. Grill chicken on a pan for 5-6 minutes on each side, or until thoroughly cooked through. Ready to serve.

Spicy Mediterranean Pasta

Total Time: 25 minutes

Servings: 8

Nutrition Facts:

Calories: 281 kcal

Total fats: 8 g

Proteins: 10 g

Carbohydrates: 45 g

Ingredients:

- 1 pkg dry whole wheat rotini
- 1 bag broccoli florets
- ¼ cup olive oil
- 4 finely chopped garlic cloves
- 14.5 oz can diced tomatoes with basil, garlic, and oregano, undrained
- 15 oz can of cannellini beans
- 2 tbsp balsamic vinegar
- ½ tsp crushed red pepper flakes
- ½ tsp salt
- ¼ tsp ground black pepper

Instructions:

1. Cook the rotini pasta according to package instructions. Add broccoli last 8 minutes of pasta cooking time.
2. Using a skillet, heat oil over medium heat. Add garlic and stir until fragrant, which will take about a minute. Carefully add the vinegar, tomatoes, beans, and red pepper. Cook for 5 minutes while stirring occasionally.
3. Drain pasta mixture, and reserve one cup of cooking water. Return pasta and broccoli to the saucepan. Add tomato mixture, salt and pepper, toss well to coat. If the pasta mixture is too dry, you can add the reserved cooking water, ½ cup at a time, to your liking. Pasta is ready to serve.

Mediterranean Calamari

Total Time: 20 minutes

Servings: 2

Nutrition Facts:

Calories: 308.8

Total fats: 25.7 g

Proteins: 1.9 g

Carbohydrates: 10.2 g

Ingredients:

- 2 tbsp roasted garlic
- 2 tbsp olive oil
- 2 cups calamari
- 2 tbsp tossed caper
- 1 tsp cumin
- 1 tsp chopped ancho chili
- 1 tsp red pepper flakes
- 2 diced medium plum tomatoes
- ½ cup white wine
- 3 tbsp lime juice
- 1 tbsp Italian parsley
- 2 tbsp unsalted
- Salt to taste

Instructions:

1. Add oil to a pan, heat on medium, add garlic and calamari.
2. Sauté for 1 minute, then add diced tomatoes, chopped ancho chili, capers, cumin, and red pepper flakes. Cook for 1 more minute.
3. Add white wine and lime juice. Let simmer for 4 minutes.
4. Add chopped parsley, salt, and butter.
5. Reduce heat until sauce thickens. It will be ready to serve. May serve with french bread if desired.

Mediterranean Pizza

Total Time: 17 minutes

Servings: 4

Nutrition Facts:

Calories: 291 kcal

Total fat: 11 g

Proteins: 14 g

Carbohydrates: 34 g

Ingredients:

- 1 12-inch prepared pizza crust
- ¼ tsp crushed red pepper
- ¼ tsp dried Italian seasoning
- 1 cup crumbled goat cheese
- 3 sliced plum tomatoes
- 6 chopped kalamata olives
- 14 oz can quartered artichoke hearts
- ¼ cup chopped fresh basil
- Olive oil to grease baking sheet

Instructions:

1. Preheat the oven to 450 degrees-F.
2. Sprinkle pizza crust with crushed red pepper and fried Italian seasoning.
3. Coat the crust evenly with the crumbled goat cheese with about ½ inch around the borders. Using a spoon, gently press the cheese down into the crust.
4. Arrange the plum tomato slices, chopped kalamata olives, and artichoke hearts on the pizza. Arrange as desired.
5. Coat baking sheet with olive oil and place pizza on top. Bake in oven for 10-12 minutes or until the crust is crisp and cheese is bubbly.

6. Sprinkle the chopped basil over the top and it is ready to serve.

You may not think of pizza as healthy, however, the fresh Mediterranean or Italian pizza with the healthy ingredients will be unlike any other pizza you have had. It is far ahead of that excessively greasy pizza you get from your local pizza parlor.

Cilantro Lime Chicken

Total time: 65 minutes

Servings: 8 pieces

Nutrition Facts:

Calories: 212 kcal

Total fats: 8.1 g

Proteins: 30.1 g

Carbohydrates: 2.8 g

Ingredients:

- 8 boneless chicken thighs with the skin on
- Extra virgin olive oil
- 6 roughly chopped garlic cloves
- 1 cup dry white wine
- Juice from 2 limes
- 2 cups chicken broth
- 1 bunch chopped cilantro

Spice mix

- 1 tbsp seasoned salt
- 1 tsp black pepper
- 1 tbsp garlic powder
- 1 tsp paprika
- ½ tsp ground nutmeg

Instructions:

1. Turn on the oven and preheat to 375 degrees-F.
2. In a saucer, mix all of the spices. Take the chicken thighs and season each side with the spice mix. Season under the skin as well and let the chicken sit for 15 minutes.
3. Using a heavy skillet, heat 1-2 tbsp olive oil. Lightly brown the chicken thighs evenly on both sides. Remove the chicken from the skillet and set aside on a plate.
4. Lower the heat on the skillet and deglaze with white wine. Allow the white wine to reduce by cooking and then add the broth.
5. Bring the liquid to a simmer, then add garlic and lime juice.
6. Return the chicken to the skillet, toss in the cilantro, bring to a simmer for about 5 minutes.
7. Cover and then transfer to the oven. Allow baking for 45 minutes, or until the chicken is cooked through.
8. Remove chicken from the oven and let sit for 5 minutes.
9. Garnish with the cilantro and it is ready to serve.

Roasted Greek Potatoes

Total Time: 65 minutes

Servings: 6

Nutrition Facts:

Calories: 409 kcal

Total fats: 8.2 g

Proteins: 13.8 g

Carbohydrates: 77 g

Ingredients:

Spice mix

- 1 tsp seasoned salt
- 1 tsp ground black pepper
- 1 tsp sweet paprika
- 1 tsp organic rosemary

Potatoes

- 4 large potatoes for baking (Peeled, washed, and cut into wedges)
- 8 large chopped garlic cloves
- 4 tbsp extra virgin olive oil
- Juice from 1 whole lemon
- 1-¼ cup vegetable broth (May use chicken broth)
- ½ cup grated parmesan cheese
- 1 cup chopped parsley leaves

Instructions:

1. Turn on the oven and preheat to 400 degrees-F.
2. Using a small saucer, mix all of the spices together and set aside.
3. Lightly grease the baking dish with oil. Place potato wedges on a baking dish and sprinkle with the spice mix. Toss potatoes to evenly distribute spices.
4. In a bowl, whisk together chopped garlic, olive oil, lemon juice, and broth. Pour this mixture into the baking dish with potatoes.
5. Cover the baking dish with foil. allow 40 minutes for baking in the oven.
6. Remove from the oven briefly, and sprinkle potato wedges with parmesan cheese. Place back into the oven uncovered and bake for another 10-15 minutes or until potatoes are cooked through. They should be a nice golden-brown color.
7. Remove from the oven, garnish with parsley and serve.

Mediterranean-Style Wine Braised Lamb Shanks With Vegetables

Total Time: 3 hours

Servings: 6

Nutrition Facts:

Calories: 301 kcal

Total fats: 9.5 g

Proteins: 20.4 g

Carbohydrates: 34.4 g

Ingredients:

Spice mix

- 2-¼ tsp garlic powder
- 1 tsp sweet paprika
- ¾ tsp ground nutmeg
- 1 tsp freshly ground black pepper
- 1 tsp salt

Lamb

- 6 lamb shanks
- 2 tbsp olive oil
- 2 chopped celery ribs
- 3 large carrots, peeled and cut into small pieces
- 1 chopped medium yellow onion
- 1 pound baby potatoes
- 2 cups dry red wine
- 3 cups low-sodium beef broth
- 28 oz can peeled tomatoes
- 2 cinnamon sticks
- 4 sprigs fresh thyme
- 2 sprigs fresh rosemary

Side

- Lebanese rice prepared according to package instructions.
- You may also use Fattoush salad as a side. See recipe in the salad section.

Instructions:

1. Preheat the oven to 350 degrees-F.
2. Add spice ingredients to a saucer and mix well to combine.
3. Pat the lamb shanks dry and season with spice mix all around.
4. Using a dutch oven, heat 2 tbsp olive oil over medium to high heat. Place just a few lamb shanks at a time to brown them evenly. Transfer the lamb shanks to a large tray or bowl. Dispose of any excess fat from the dutch oven pot.
5. Add the onions, celery, carrots, and potatoes. Saute on medium heat for 5-7 minutes. The vegetables should gain some color by now. Add the wine and scrape up all of the brown bits in the pot. Cook briefly so the wine reduces in amount a little bit.
6. Add the broth, tomatoes, cinnamon sticks, thyme, and rosemary. Sprinkle some salt and pepper. Return lamb shanks to the dutch oven. Submerge into the liquid, and let boil for 10 minutes. Turn the heat off at this time.
7. Cover the dutch oven and transfer to the oven. Cook for 2.5 hours. Check the pot periodically while cooking just in case you need to add more liquid.
8. After cooking, the liquid should have reduced to ⅓ of the original amount.
9. You may prepare the side according to their own instructions while lamb shanks are cooking.
10. Serve the lamb shanks with the sides and enjoy.

Mujadara: Lebanese Rice With Lentils

Total Time: 82 minutes

Servings: 4-6

Nutrition Facts:

Calories: 405 kcal

Total fats: 16.9 g

Proteins: 10.9 g

Carbohydrates: 52.4 g

Ingredients:

- 1 cup black lentils, rinsed
- 4 cups of water
- ¼ cup extra virgin olive oil
- 2 large diced yellow onions
- 1 tsp kosher salt, may add more to taste
- 1 cup long-grain white rice, soaked in water for 10-15 minutes and then drained
- Freshly ground black pepper
- Parsley for garnish

Instructions:

1. Add 2 cups of water and lentils to a saucepan. Turn on high heat and bring water to a boil. Once boiling, reduce heat and let simmer. Cover the pan and let boil for 10-12 minutes. Drain the lentils carefully and set aside.
2. In a large sauté pan with a lid, heat the oil using medium to high heat. Add the diced onions and cook until dark golden brown. Sprinkle the onions with a teaspoon of salt as they cook.
3. Pour 2 cups of water and boil on high heat, then reduce heat to low and simmer for 2 minutes. Stir the rice and lentils into the onion mix. Cover and bring back to a boil.
4. Stir in a pinch of salt and pepper. Reduce heat to low and cover. Cook until the liquid has been absorbed and the rice and lentils are cooked through. This will take 20 minutes.

5. Turn off the heat and sprinkle with salt and pepper for flavoring. Drizzle the mujadara with extra virgin olive oil and garnish with parsley. It is ready to serve.

Chorizo Pilaf

Total Time: 50 minutes

Servings: 4

Nutrition Facts:

Calories: 488 kcal

Total Fats: 18 g

Protein: 19 g

Carbohydrates: 58 g

Ingredients:

- 1 large thinly sliced onion
- 1 tbsp olive oil
- 250 g baby chorizo, sliced
- 4 crushed garlic cloves
- 400 g chopped tomatoes
- 1 tsp smoked paprika
- 250 g basmati rice
- 600 ml vegetable stock
- 1 lemon zest, plus wedges for serving
- Small bunch of parsley, chopped
- 2 fresh bay leaves

Instructions:

1. Using a large pan, heat olive oil on medium. Add in the onions and cook for 5-8 minutes until soft and golden.
2. Push onions to one side of the pan and add chorizo. Cook until lightly brown and some of the oils are released into the pan.

3. Add garlic, paprika, and then the tomatoes. Bubble over medium heat for 5 minutes. Add the rice, stock, lemon zest, and bay leaves.
4. Stir everything together and bring to a boil. Cover with a lid and cook on the lowest heat for 12 minutes.
5. Turn off heat and let sit and steam for 10-15 minutes. Stir in the parsley and serve with lemon wedges to squeeze over chorizo.

Mediterranean Stuffed Tomatoes

Total Time: 20 minutes

Servings: 4

Nutrition Facts:

Calories: 132 kcal

Total Fats: 4 g

Proteins: 5 g

Carbohydrates: 21 g

Ingredients:

- 4 medium ripe tomatoes
- 1 cup cooked quinoa (or brown rice)
- ½ cup no-salt-added cannellini beans, canned
- ⅓ cup torn fresh basil leaves
- 1 tsp olive oil
- 1 oz crumbled feta cheese
- ¼ tsp black pepper
- ⅛ tsp kosher salt

Instructions:

1. Preheat oven to 375 degrees-F.
2. Cut the tops off tomatoes and discard.
3. Carefully scoop out the pulp. Leave the shells intact and reserve ½ cup of pulp.
4. Finely chop the reserved pulp.

5. Place the tomato shells in a small square dish.
6. Mix the rice, chopped tomato pulp, beans, feta, basil, oil, pepper, and salt in a large basin until combined well. Divide mixture evenly among the tomato shells.
7. Bake for about 12 minutes.
8. Take out the oven and they are ready to serve.

Mediterranean Snapper Tray Bake

Total Time: 85 minutes

Servings: 8

Nutrition Facts:

Calories: 359 kcal

Total fats: 11.5 g

Proteins: 42.3 g

Carbohydrates: 16.1 g

Ingredients:

- 400 g cherry truss tomatoes
- 2 tbsp lemon juice
- ⅔ cup dry white wine
- 4 crushed garlic cloves
- 2 tsp ground coriander
- 1 tsp sweet paprika
- ⅔ cup extra virgin olive oil
- 1 kg red-skinned potatoes, cut into small cubes
- ⅔ cup fresh dill sprigs
- ⅔ cup fresh oregano leaves
- 2 tsp lemon rind
- 1 tsp caraway seeds
- 1.5 kg whole snapper, cleaned
- ⅓ cup kalamata olives
- 2 tbsp drained capers
- lemon wedges for serving

Instructions:

1. Preheat the oven to 400 degrees-F.
2. Grease a large baking tray with oil.
3. Place half of the tomatoes in a bowl, crush with your hands.
4. Add wine, lemon juice, garlic, coriander, paprika, and 1 tbsp olive oil.
5. Season with salt and pepper. Stir everything to combine.
6. Add potato and toss to combine.
7. Place potato mixture on the prepared tray and bake for 30 minutes.
8. While baking, place oregano, dill, rind, caraway seeds, and remaining oil in a small food processor. Season with salt and pepper. Process until finely chopped.
9. Make 4 slits on each side of the snapper fish. Rub dill mixture in cavity and slits of fish.
10. Place fish onto potato mixture and bake another 15 minutes.
11. Cut remaining tomatoes into small portions. Add tomatoes, olives, and capers to tray in the oven. Bake for another 15 minutes or until fish is cooked through.
12. Sprinkle with the herbs and serve with the lemon wedges.

Salmon Skewer With Caper and Dill Butter Sauce

Total Time: 20 minutes

Servings: 4

Nutrition Facts:

Calories: 640 kcal

Total Fats: 32.4 g

Proteins: 26.8 g

Carbohydrates: 70 g

Ingredients:

- 400 g of skinless and boneless salmon, cut into 2 cm pieces
- 250 g mini Roma tomatoes
- 1 yellow bell pepper, cut into 2 cm pieces
- 1 tsp lemon pepper seasoning
- ¼ cup extra virgin olive oil
- 1 tbsp drained capers
- 50 g chopped butter
- 2 tbsp grated lemon peel
- ⅓ cup lemon juice
- ¼ cup fresh dill leaves

Instructions:

1. To start, you will need 8 pre-soaked bamboo skewers.
2. Thread salmon, bell pepper, and tomato onto skewers.
3. Brush 1 tbsp oil and then sprinkle with lemon pepper
4. Take the remainder of oil and heat on high in a small saucepan. Add capers and then cook for 1-2 minutes or until they are crisp, not brown.
5. Reduce heat to low. Stir in the butter until melted and foamy.
6. Remove pan from heat, stir in lemon peel, lemon juice, and dill. Season with salt and pepper. Cover for now to keep warm.
7. Heat chargrill pan on medium to high heat. Cook skewers while occasionally turning for 4 minutes.
8. Serve with rice or baby spinach.

One-Skillet Mediterranean Chicken Recipe With Tomatoes and Green Olives

Total Time: 25 minutes

Servings: 4

Nutrition Facts:

Calories: 135 kcal

Total Fats: 5.8 g

Proteins: 9.6 g

Carbohydrates: 12.1 g

Ingredients:

- 4 boneless and skinless chicken breasts of equal size
- Salt and pepper
- 1 tbsp dried oregano
- 2 tbsp garlic paste
- Extra virgin olive oil
- ½ dry white wine
- Juice from 1 lemon
- ½ cup chicken broth
- 1 cup chopped red onion
- 1 ½ cup diced tomatoes
- ¼ cup sliced green olives
- A handful of chopped fresh parsley
- Optional crumbled feta cheese

Instructions:

1. Pat the chicken dry using a paper towel.
2. Make three slits through on each side of the chicken breasts.
3. Spread the garlic on both sides and insert some into the slits.
4. Sprinkle both sides of the chicken breasts with pepper, salt, and oregano for seasoning.
5. In a large cast-iron skillet, heat 2 tbsp olive oil on medium. Brown the chicken on both sides.
6. Add white wine and cook to reduce by ½, then add lemon juice and chicken broth. Sprinkle the remaining oregano on top.

7. Reduce heat slightly to low-medium. Cover with a lid and cook for 10-15 minutes. Turn the chicken over once during this time.
8. Uncover and top with onions, tomatoes, and olives. Cover once more and cook for 3 minutes.
9. Lastly, add feta cheese and parsley on top.
10. Serve with light pasta, rice or couscous.

Easy Italian Baked Chicken

Total Time: 28 minutes

Servings: 6

Nutrition Facts:

Calories: 290 kcal

Total Fats: 11.5 g

Proteins: 35.9 g

Carbohydrates: 11 g

Ingredients:

- 2 pounds boneless and skinless chicken breast
- 2 tsp oregano
- 1 tsp fresh thyme
- 1 tsp sweet paprika
- salt and pepper to taste
- 4 minced garlic cloves
- 3 tbsp extra virgin olive oil
- Juice from 1 lemon
- 1 medium red onion, thinly sliced
- 6 small roma tomatoes, halved
- Handful of chopped fresh parsley
- Fresh basil leaves

Instructions:

1. Preheat your oven to 425 degrees-F.

2. Pat the chicken dry and then place it in a large zip top bag. Release any air from the bag before you zip it. Place it on your poultry cutting board. Pound the chicken flat using a meat mallet. Do this for each chicken breast one at a time.
3. Sprinkle pepper and salt on both sides of chicken and place in a large mixing bowl.
4. Add the spices, garlic, lemon juice, and olive oil. Combine to make sure the chicken is evenly coated.
5. In a large baking dish, lightly oil it and then spread the onions on the bottom. Arrange seasoned chicken on top and add the tomatoes.
6. Cover the baking dish lightly with foil and bake for 10 minutes. Using an instant meat thermometer, ensure internal chicken temperature 165 degrees.
7. Remove from heat, let chicken breasts rest covered for 5-10 minutes. Uncover and garnish with parsley and basil.

Breakfast

I will now provide some delicious breakfast recipes common in Mediterranean cuisine. These will be a delicious and healthy way to begin each and every morning.

Shakshuka

Total Time: 30 minutes

Servings: 4

Nutrition Facts:

Calories: 179 kcal

Total fats: 11 g

Proteins: 7 g

Carbohydrates: 12 g

Ingredients:

- 2 tablespoons of olive oil
- 1 finely chopped yellow onion
- 2 finely sliced red bell peppers
- 2 cloves garlic
- 15 oz can of chopped tomatoes
- 1 tsp sugar
- 1 tsp spicy harissa
- 4 eggs
- 1 tbsp chopped parsley
- Salt to taste
- Freshly ground black pepper to taste

Instructions:

1. Heat oil in a heavy cast-iron skillet. Heat the oil in a heavy skillet.
2. Add the onions and peppers, cook for about 5 minutes, until soft.
3. Cook 1 more minute after adding garlic.
4. Add tomatoes, sugar, and harissa and then cook for about 7 minutes.
5. Season with the salt and pepper to taste. You may also add more harissa for extra spice level.
6. With a wooden spoon, make 4 indentations in the mixture. Add egg into each mark.
7. Cover the pot and cook until the egg whites are getting set.
8. Sprinkle fresh parsley and it is now ready to serve. Enjoy with pita bread.

Breakfast Sandwich

Total Time: 20 minutes

Servings: 4

Nutrition Facts:

Calories: 242

Total fats: 12 g

Proteins: 13 g

Carbohydrates: 25 g

Ingredients:

- 4 multigrain sandwich thins
- 4 tsp olive oil
- 4 eggs
- 1 tbsp fresh rosemary
- 2 cups fresh baby spinach leaves
- 1 medium tomato, cut into 8 slices
- Pinch of kosher salt
- Freshly ground black pepper to taste

Instructions:

1. Turn on the oven and preheat 375 degrees-F.
2. Split the sandwich thins. Brush the cut sides with 2 tsp olive oil and place on a baking sheet. Toast in the oven for about 5 minutes or until the edges are lightly brown.
3. In a large skillet, heat the remaining 2 tsp olive oil and rosemary over high heat. Break and place whole eggs one at a time into the skillet. The yolk should still be runny, but the egg whites should be set.
4. Break yolks up with a spatula. Flip the egg and cook on other side until done. Remove eggs from heat.
5. Place bottom halves of toasted sandwich thins on medium on 4 separate plates. Divine spinach among the thins.
6. Top each thin with two tomato slices, cooked egg, and 1 tbsp of feta cheese.
7. Lightly sprinkle with salt and pepper for flavoring. Place remaining sandwich thin halves over the top and they are ready to serve.

Breakfast Burrito

Total Time: 20 minutes

Servings: 6

Nutrition Facts:

Calories: 252 kcal

Total fats: 11 g

Proteins: 14 g

Carbohydrates: 21 g

Ingredient:

- 6 tortillas of your choice-whole 10 inches
- 9 eggs
- 2 cups baby spinach
- 3 tbsp sliced black olives
- 3 tbsp chopped sun-dried tomatoes
- ½ cup feta cheese
- ¾ cup canned refried beans

Instructions:

1. Spray medium saucepan with cooking spray.
2. Scramble eggs on medium heat and toss for about 5 minutes. Eggs should no longer be liquid. Add spinach, black olives, sun-dried tomatoes, and continue to stir and toss until no longer wet.
3. Add feta cheese and cover until melted.
4. Add 2 tbsp refried beans to each tortilla. Top with egg mixture evenly between all 6 tortillas. Wrap them up like a burrito.
5. Grill on a panini press until lightly brown. You may also use a frying pan if no press available.
6. You may add a salsa of your choice if you wish to do so.

Breakfast Couscous

Total Time: 8 minutes

Servings: 4

Nutrition Facts:

Calories: 306 kcal

Total fats: 6 g

Proteins: 11 g

Carbohydrates: 55 g

Ingredients:

- 3 cups of low-fat milk
- 1 cup uncooked whole-wheat couscous
- 1 cinnamon stick
- ½ chopped dried apricot
- ¼ cup dried currants
- 6 tsp brown sugar
- ¼ tsp salt
- 4 tsp butter, melted and divided

Instructions:

1. Take a large saucepan and combine milk and cinnamon stick and heat over medium.
2. Heat 3 minutes or until microbubbles form around edges of the pan. Do not boil.
3. Remove from heat, stir in the couscous, apricots, currants, salt, and 4 tsp brown sugar. Cover the mixture and allow it to sit for 15 minutes. Remove and throw away the cinnamon stick.
4. Divide couscous among 4 bowls, and top each with 1 tsp melted butter and ½ tsp brown sugar. Ready to serve.

Breakfast Egg Muffins

Total Time: 40 minutes

Servings: 12 muffins

Nutrition Facts:

Calories: 67 kcal

Total Fats: 4.7 g

Proteins: 4.6 g

Carbohydrates: 1.2 g

Ingredients:

- Extra virgin olive oil for brushing
- 1 small chopped red bell pepper
- 1 finely chopped shallot
- 10 pitted and chopped kalamata olives
- 4 oz cooked chicken or turkey, boneless and shredded
- 1 oz chopped fresh parsley leaves
- 8 large eggs
- Salt and pepper to taste
- Handful of crumbled feta
- ½ tsp paprika
- ¼ tsp ground turmeric

Instructions:

1. Preheat to 350 degrees-F.
2. Prepare a 12-cup muffin pan by brushing with olive oil.
3. Divide the peppers, tomatoes, shallots, olives, chicken or turkey, parsley, and crumbled feta evenly among the 12 cups.
4. In a large mixing bowl, add eggs, spices, salt, and pepper. Whisk well to combine.
5. Pour the egg mixture over each cup in the muffin pan, leaving a little bit of room at the top. Each cup should be about ¾ of the way full.

6. Place muffin pan on top of a sheet pan. Bake in the oven for 25 minutes or until egg muffins are set.
7. Let cool for a few minutes and then remove egg muffins by gently using a butter knife first to loosen. They are now ready to serve.

Baked Eggs With Pistou

Total Time: 15 minutes

Servings: 2

Nutrition Facts:

Calories: 310 kcal

Total fats: 22 g

Proteins: 4 g

Carbohydrates: 30 g

Ingredients:

- 4 organic eggs
- ¼ cup of cooked white beans
- ½ cup of diced tomatoes
- Tomato spice blend
- Pistou-basil, parmesan, fresh garlic, olive oil, salt.

Instructions:

1. Rinse the white beans.
2. Warm up 2 tsp olive oil in a medium frying pan over medium to high heat, until hot, but not smoking.
3. Add the tomatoes, tomato spice paste, 2 tbsp water and season with salt and pepper.
4. Cook, while stirring occasionally, until the sauce thickens, which will take 3 to 5 minutes.
5. Stir in the beans.
6. Crack the eggs into the pan of tomato sauce and season with salt and pepper. Cover and cook until

white part of the eggs set but the yolks are still runny. Will take about 6-8 minutes.
7. Transfer the eggs and tomato sauce to individual plates and drizzle with the pistou. Ready to serve.

Salads

There are many terrific salads that are part of Mediterranean cuisine. They are loaded with ingredients and very nutrient-dense. These are unlike any salads you have ever had before and can actually be meals all by themselves. We will detail some of the most popular ones in this diet plan.

Mediterranean Orzo Salad

Total Time: 1 hour 25 minutes

Servings: 12

Nutrition Facts:

Calories: 260

Total Fats: 10 g

Proteins: 9 g

Carbohydrates: 36 g

Ingredients:

- ¼ cup extra virgin olive oil
- Juice from 1 lemon
- 1 Minced garlic clove
- ½ diced purple onion
- Ground black pepper to taste
- 12 orzo pasta, cooked, drained, and cooled
- Salt to taste
- 1 cup cherry tomatoes
- 1 cup of yellow grapes (substitute with an additional cup of cherry tomatoes)
- 1 cup crumbled feta cheese
- 1 cup of halved kalamata olives

- 1 cup garbanzo beans
- 3 tbsp minced parsley

Instructions:

1. Cook the orzo pasta according to package instructions.
2. In a bowl, mix together the garlic, olive oil, lemon juice, pepper, and salt until totally combined.
3. Place the orzo and all other ingredients in a large mixing bowl and then pour the dressing from the previous step over the top.
4. Stir and combine everything well. May add extra seasonings according to your taste.
5. Add more feta and parsley on top and it is ready to serve.

Mediterranean Couscous Salad

Total Time: 30 minutes

Servings: 6

Nutrition Facts:

Calories: 231 kcal

Total fats: 12 g

Proteins:6 g

Carbohydrates: 24 g

Ingredients:

Dressing

- 4 tbsp freshly squeezed lemon juice
- 2 tbsp olive oil
- 1 tbsp white wine vinegar
- 1 tbsp Italian dressing
- 2 cloves of minced garlic
- 1 tsp sugar
- ½ tsp salt may add more to taste

- 1 tsp pepper, may add more to taste

Salad

- ¾ cup couscous, uncooked
- 1 tbsp butter
- 1 English chopped cucumber
- 1 cup halved cherry tomatoes
- ½ cup sliced kalamata olives
- 1 chopped green pepper
- ½ chopped medium red onion
- ¾ cup of crumbled feta cheese
- 3 tbsp chopped fresh mint

Instructions:

1. Prepare the couscous according to package instructions.
2. Add the butter to the couscous when you're preparing. Let it cool down.
3. In a small bowl add all of the dressing ingredients and whisk well. You may also put ingredients in a jar and then shake thoroughly.
4. To a large bowl, add the prepared couscous and fluff it up with a fork.
5. Add the remainder of salad ingredients. Pour the dressing over the top and toss everything together well.

Fattoush Salad

Total Time: 20 minutes

Servings: 6

Nutrition Facts:

Calories: 345 kcal

Total fats: 20.4 g

Proteins: 9.1 g

Carbohydrates: 39.8 g

Ingredients:

- Extra virgin olive oil
- ½ tsp sumac (spice from a sumac flower)
- Ground black pepper to taste
- Salt to taste
- 1 heart of romaine lettuce, chopped
- 1 chopped English cucumber
- 5 chopped Roma tomatoes
- 5 whole green onions, chopped
- 5 radishes thinly chopped, with their stems removed
- 2 cups chopped fresh parsley
- 1 cup chopped fresh mint leaves
- 2 loaves pita bread

Lime vinaigrette

- Juice from 1 ½ limes
- ⅓ cup of extra virgin olive oil
- salt and pepper to taste
- 1 tsp ground sumac
- ¼ tsp ground cinnamon
- ¼ tsp ground allspice

Instructions:

1. Toast pita bread in the toaster oven until crisp.
2. Heat 3 tsps olive oil in a large pan. You can fry pita bread in the large circles and break apart afterwards with the end of a whisk or spatula, or break into small strips before frying as we do here. Toss the bread pieces frequently, until lightly brown on both sides.
3. Add salt, pepper, and ½ tsp sumac. Remove pita chips from heat and place them on a paper towel to drain.
4. In a large mixing bowl, combine the cucumber, tomatoes, chopped lettuce, green onions, sliced radish, and parsley.
5. For lime vinaigrette, whisk together lime juice, olive oil, and spices in a small bowl.

6. Dress the salad with the dressing and toss lightly.
7. Add the pita chips and toss with more sumac if you prefer, and transfer to a small mixing bowl.

Mediterranean Steak Bowls

Total Time: 45 minutes

Servings: 4

Nutrition Facts:

Calories: 513 kcal

Total fats: 28 g

Proteins: 37 g

Carbohydrates: 28 g

Ingredients:

Bowls

- 1 pound flank steak
- 1 pint cherry tomatoes
- ½ peeled and cut medium red onion
- 1 chopped head of romaine lettuce
- 1 large chopped cucumber
- ⅓ cup sliced pitted kalamata olives
- 1 cup of hummus, the flavor of your choice
- ½ cup crumbled feta cheese
- Skewers for the veggies
- 2 tsp of avocado oil
- lemon wedges for garnish

Herbed-yogurt dressing

- 1 cup of plain yogurt
- 1 tbsp avocado oil
- Juice from half a lemon
- 1 large minced garlic clove

- ½ tsp dried oregano
- ½ tsp dried dill
- ½ tsp salt
- 2 tsp dried fresh mint

Instructions:

Dressing

1. Take all of the dressing ingredients and place them in a small bowl. Whisk well to combine. Store in the fridge until ready to use, maximum 5 days.

Bowls

1. Preheat grill to high heat, around 450 degrees-F.
2. After patting the steak dry, sprinkle both sides with salt and pepper.
3. Thread the cherry tomatoes and quarter cut onions through the skewers, brush with oil, sprinkle salt and pepper.
4. When the grill is hot, place flank steak and tomato skewer on the grill. Turn the veggies occasionally. Cook for 5-8 minutes or until onions are softened. Tomatoes will also blister.
5. Grill the steak for 4-5 minutes on each side. This will make it medium rare. May cook an extra 1-2 minutes on each side if desired.
6. Remove steak to a plate and cover loosely for 10 minutes. Then slice thinly against the grain.
7. Divide chopped romaine between 4 plates. Top with sliced steak, grilled vegetables, hummus, chopped cucumbers, olives, and feta cheese.
8. Drizzle the dressing we made earlier. Garnish with lemon wedges and it is ready to serve.

Tabouli Salad

Total Time: 20 minutes

Servings: 6-8

Nutrition Facts:

Calories: 190 kcal

Total fats: 10 g

Proteins: 3.2 g

Carbohydrates: 25.5 g

Ingredients:

- ½ cup bulgur wheat
- 4 finely chopped Roma tomatoes
- 1 chopped English cucumber
- 12-15 fresh mint leaves, finely chopped
- Salt to taste
- 4 tbsp extra virgin olive oil
- 4 tbsp lime juice
- Romaine lettuce leaves for serving (optional)

Instructions:

1. Wash the bulgar wheat and soak in water for 5-7 minutes. Drain well and also squeeze bulgur by hand to get out excess water.
2. Finely chop all of the vegetables, herbs and green onions and place them in a bowl. Add the bulgur and sprinkle with salt for flavoring. Mix gently.
3. Add lime juice and olive oil and mix once more.
4. Cover the tabouli salad and refrigerate for 30 minutes to get the best results. Serve the tabouli by itself or on top of the Romaine leaves. You may also use pita bread if desired.

Greek Salad

Total Time: 10 minutes

Servings: 3

Nutrition Facts:

Calories: 372 kcal

Total fats: 29 g

Proteins: 10 g

Carbohydrates: 23 g

Ingredients:

- ¼ cup extra virgin olive oil
- 2 tbsp red wine vinegar
- 1 large cucumber, chopped
- ½ cup kalamata olives
- ½ tsp salt
- ½ tsp ground black pepper
- 1 tsp dried oregano
- 4 large sliced tomatoes
- 1 large sliced onion
- 4 cups chopped romaine lettuce (or lettuce of choice)
- 4 oz crumbled feta cheese
- 1 lemon zest

Instructions:

1. In a small saucer, mix the vinegar, olive oil, salt and pepper. This will be your dressing for later.
2. In a salad bowl, mix all of the vegetables, feta cheese, lemon zest, and dried oregano.
3. Add the dressing over the top, toss and mix everything together well. This is a very basic Greek salad.

Mediterranean Potato Salad

Total Time: 35 minutes

Servings: 4

Nutrition Facts:

Calories: 111 kcal

Total Fats: 4 g

Proteins: 3 g

Carbohydrates: 16 g

Ingredients:

- 1 tbsp olive oil
- 1 crushed garlic clove
- 1 thinly sliced yellow onion
- 1 tsp fresh oregano (May use dried)
- 100 g roasted red pepper, sliced
- 200 g can cherry tomatoes
- 300 g new potatoes, halved if large
- 25 g sliced black olives
- A handful of basil leaves, torn

Instructions:

1. Heat olive oil in a saucepan on medium heat. Add onion and cook for 5-10 minutes until soft. Add garlic and oregano and cook for another minute.
2. Add tomatoes and pepper, season well and let simmer for 10 minutes.
3. Cook the potatoes in boiling water for 10-15 minutes. Advised to add salt to water for improved cooking and tenderness. Drain and mix with the sauce made previously.
4. Sprinkle olives and basil and it's ready to serve.

Chopped Salad With Oregano Vinaigrette

Total Time: 45 minutes

Servings: 6

Nutrition Facts:

Calories: 423 kcal

Total Fats: 26.8 g

proteins: 12.9 g

Carbohydrates: 35.6

Ingredients:

Dressing

- 3 cloves of minced garlic
- ¼ cup red wine vinegar
- 1 tbsp dried oregano
- ½ tsp dijon mustard
- 1 tsp kosher salt
- Freshly ground black pepper
- ½ cup extra virgin olive oil

Salad

- ½ cup farro, pearled
- 1tsp kosher salt
- 2 medium bell peppers
- 2 large stalks of celery
- ½ medium English cucumber
- ½ small red onion
- 8 small pickled pepperoncinis
- 6 oz feta cheese, cut into cubes
- 15 oz can of chickpeas

Serving

- ½ head of an iceberg lettuce
- 1 head radicchio (Chicory)

Instructions:

1. For vinaigrette, place 3 minced garlic cloves in a large bowl. Add ¼ cup red wine vinegar, 1 tbsp oregano, 1 tsp kosher salt, ½ tsp dijon mustard, several grinds of black pepper, and then whisk to combine.

2. While whisking, slowly drizzle the ½ cup olive oil until it is emulsified.
3. Pour half of the dressing into a sealed container and place in the refrigerator for later.
4. Set aside the bowl of remaining vinaigrette.
5. To make the salad: Place ½ cup farro in a fine-mesh strainer, rinse under cool water, and then allow to drain.
6. Boil 6 cups of water in a saucepan over medium to high heat.
7. Stir in the farro and kosher salt. Boil until farro is tender, which will take about 15 minutes. Drain and then return to saucepan.
8. In the bowl of vinaigrette add the following after preparing: Core, seed, and dice 2 bell peppers, 2 large celery stalks, ½ cucumber, thinly slice red onion into half-moons, slice 8 small pepperoncinis, cut 6 oz feta cheese into small cubes, drain and rinse the chickpeas.
9. Add the farro to the dressing bowl and toss to combine. If needed, add more salt to your taste.
10. Core and chop the iceberg lettuce head into small strips. Core and chop 1 radicchio into small strips. Transfer both of these to a large airtight container and toss to combine. Refrigerate if not ready to eat yet.
11. When you are ready to eat, take equal amounts of chickpea and lettuce mixture and toss together. If the salad is too dry for you, you may add the reserve vinaigrette dressing from the fridge.

Lemon Herb Mediterranean Chicken Salad

Total Time: 25 minutes

Servings: 4

Nutrition Facts:

Calories: 336 kcal

Total fats: 21 g

Proteins: 24 g

Carbohydrates: 13 g

Ingredients:

Dressing

- Juice of 1 lemon
- 2 tbsp olive oil
- 2 tbsp water
- 2 tbsp red wine vinegar
- 2 tbsp fresh chopped parsley
- 2 tsp dried basil
- 2 tsp minced garlic
- 1 tsp dried oregano
- Cracked black pepper to taste
- 1 tsp salt
- 1 pound skinless and boneless chicken breasts

Salad

- 4 cups romaine lettuce leaves
- 1 large diced cucumber
- 2 diced Roma tomatoes
- 1 sliced red onion
- 1 sliced avocado
- Lemon wedges for serving

Instructions:

1. Take all of the ingredients for the dressing and whisk together in a large jug. Pour out half and place in the refrigerator for dressing later.
2. Set aside the remaining dressing in a bowl.
3. Add the chicken to the dressing to marinade for 15-30 minutes. In the meantime, thoroughly combine all of the salad ingredients in a large bowl.
4. Once the chicken is ready, heat 1 tbsp of oil in a grill pan over medium-high heat and grill both sides of chicken until browned and cooked through.

5. Allow chicken to cool for 5 minutes, slice and arrange as desired over salad. Drizzle with the untouched dressing. Serve with lemon wedges.

Soups

Mediterranean cuisine boasts many delicious and hearty soups that are chalk full of nutrients. You will love these soups as they will fill you up and make you smile. Just like with the salads, these soups can be used as a side, or as meals of their own.

Mediterranean-Style Homemade Vegetable Soup

Total Time: 45 minutes

Servings: 6

Nutrition Facts:

Calories: 140 kcal

Total Fats: 3.7 g

Proteins: 5.4 g

Carbohydrates: 24.3 g

Ingredients:

- 8 oz sliced baby mushrooms
- Extra virgin olive oil
- 1 bunch flat-leaf parsley
- 1 medium-sized yellow onion, chopped
- 2 chopped garlic cloves
- 2 chopped celery ribs
- 2 peeled and chopped carrots
- 2 medium zucchinis with the tops removed, cut into half-moons or diced
- 2 peeled golden potatoes cut into cubes
- 1 tsp ground coriander
- ½ tsp turmeric powder

- ½ tsp dried thyme
- ½ tsp sweet paprika
- Salt and pepper to taste
- 32 oz can whole peeled tomatoes
- 15 oz can chickpeas
- 2 bay leaves
- 6 cups low-sodium vegetable or chicken broth
- 1 lime zest
- Juice from 1 lime
- ⅓ cup toasted pine nuts

Instructions:

1. Heat 1 tbsp olive oil in a large pot over medium-high heat until simmering. Add the mushrooms and cook for 3-5 minutes.
2. Remove from pot and set aside to rest.
3. Add more olive oil (if needed) and heat. Add the chopped parsley, onions, garlic, celery, carrots, zucchini, and diced potatoes.
4. Stir in the various spices and season with salt and pepper. Cook for about 7 minutes while stirring regularly until vegetables are soft.
5. Add the bay leaves, tomatoes, chickpeas, and broth. Bring to a boil, cook for 5 minutes then turn down to medium. Cover partially and cook for 15 minutes.
6. Add sautéed mushrooms and cook for a few more minutes until mushrooms are warmed. Stir in the parsley leaves, lime zest, and juice.
7. Take off the stove. Don't forget to remove bay leaves! Transfer soup to serving bowls and top with the (optional) pine nuts.
8. Enjoy this soup with your favorite hearty bread or pita.

White Bean Soup

Total Time: 50 minutes

Servings: 4

Nutrition Facts:

Calories: 342.4 kcal

Total Fats: 4.2 g

Proteins: 19.1 g

Carbohydrates: 59.5 g

Ingredients:

- 1 medium potato peeled and cut into cubes
- 1 large carrot peeled and diced into small pieces
- 4 cups vegetable broth
- 1 tbsp olive oil
- 1 chopped medium onion
- 3 minced garlic cloves
- 2 cups of cooked cannellini beans
- ½ tsp dried thyme
- ¼ tsp dried rosemary
- Salt and ground black pepper to taste
- 1 teaspoon lemon juice

Instructions:

1. In a large saucepan, add 2 cups of broth and bring to a boil on high heat.
2. Add the potatoes and carrots, reduce the heat, and allow to simmer for 15 minutes.
3. In the meantime, place oil in a dutch oven over medium heat, then add the onions and reduce heat to low. Cover the pot and cook for 10 minutes while occasionally stirring.
4. Add the garlic and cook for another minute. Add another cup of broth and bring to a boil.
5. Add the potatoes, carrots and their leftover liquid from cooking. Add in the thyme and rosemary and stir.
6. In a blender, place beans and the last cup of broth and puree the beans.
7. Add to the soup mixture and bring to a boil.

8. Season with salt and pepper to taste. You may add additional broth if desired to reduce thickness. Otherwise, stir in the lemon juice and enjoy.
9. May add croutons for garnish.

Mediterranean Cabbage Soup

Total Time: 30 minutes

Servings: 6

Nutrition Facts:

Calories: 205 kcal

 Total Fats: 5.5 g

Proteins: 6.2 g

Carbohydrates: 31 g

Ingredients:

- 1 cup chopped carrots
- 1 cup sliced fennel
- ½ cup chopped onion
- 2 tsp minced garlic
- 2 tbsp extra virgin olive oil
- ½ tsp ground coriander
- ½ tsp salt
- 6 cups low-sodium chicken broth
- 15 oz can of diced tomatoes, no-salt-added, with basil, garlic, and oregano
- 1 chopped head of green cabbage
- 15 oz can unsalted cannellini beans
- 2 tsp sugar
- 1 tsp fresh oregano
- Lemon zest for the garnish

Instructions:

1. In a large pot, heat the oil on medium-high heat. Add fennel, onions, and carrots. Cook while stirring occasionally for 5 minutes until the veggies start to soften.
2. Add salt, garlic, and coriander. Cook for about 1 minute until fragrant, stirring continuously.
3. Add broth and tomatoes, bring to a boil. Add cabbage and reduce heat to medium. Cook for 20 to 25 minutes until cabbage is tender, stirring occasionally.
4. Stir in the beans, sugar, and oregano. Cook for 3 minutes until the beans are heated through.
5. Sprinkle lemon zest and it is ready to serve.

Bean Soup

Total Time: 3 hours

Servings: 4

Nutrition Facts:

Calories: 189 kcal

Total fats: 5 g

Proteins: 15 g

Carbohydrates: 11 g

Ingredients:

- 1 large chopped onion
- 2 medium chopped carrots
- 1 large crushed garlic clove
- 2 cups of beans
- 8 cups water
- 1 tbsp thyme
- 1 bay leaf
- ¼ cup fresh chopped parsley
- Salt to taste
- Freshly ground black pepper to taste
- 1 tbsp extra virgin olive oil.

Instructions:

1. In a heavy soup kettle, heat the extra virgin olive oil on medium heat. Sauté onions, carrots, and garlic until they are soft but not browned. This will take about 15 minutes.
2. Add the regular beans and boiling water to the soup kettle, then add thyme, bay leaves, and parsley.
3. Cover and cook over low heat, and add boiling water as needed. Cook 1 ½-3 hours or until the beans are soft. Cooking times vary based on the age of beans.
4. When beans are soft and salt and pepper to taste.
5. Transfer soup to individual bowls.
6. Garnish with parsley and croutons if desired and drizzle with olive oil.
7. For thicker soups, you can take out some of the beans and puree in the food processor and then return them to pot. For thinner soups, you can add some extra hot water.

Mediterranean Chicken Soup

Total Time: 65 minutes

Servings: 8

Nutrition Facts:

Calories: 285 kcal

Total Fats: 5 g

Proteins: 25 g

Carbohydrates: 31 g

Ingredients:

- 1 ½ pound boneless chicken breast, cut into small cubes

- 1 tsp black pepper
- 1 tbsp Greek seasoning
- 1 tbsp olive oil
- 4 thinly sliced green onions
- 1 minced garlic clove
- ¼ cup white wine, or may use chicken broth
- 7 cups low-sodium chicken broth
- ¼ cup chopped tomatoes, sun-dried
- 1 tbsp capers
- 1 ½ tsp minced fresh basil
- 1 ½ tsp minced fresh oregano
- 1 ½ cups uncooked orzo pasta
- 2 tbsp lemon juice
- 1 ½ tsp minced fresh parsley

Instructions:

1. Season chicken with pepper and Greek seasoning.
2. Sauté the chicken in a dutch oven in oil until no longer pink. Remove and set aside.
3. Add the green onions and garlic to the pan, sauté for 1 minute. Add the white wine, stir to loosen brown bits from the pan
4. Stir in the broth, olives, capers, tomatoes, basil, oregano, and chicken. Bring to a boil.
5. Reduce heat, cover and simmer for 15 minutes and then return to a boil.
6. Stir in the orzo pasta and cook 8-10 minutes until pasta is tender.
7. Stir in the lemon juice and parsley and it is ready to serve.

Kale, Cannellini and Farro Stew

Total Time: 60 minutes

Servings: 6

Nutrition Facts:

Calories: 329 kcal

Total Fats: 8 g

Proteins: 12 g

Carbohydrates: 52 g

Ingredients:

- 2 tbsp olive oil
- 1 cup chopped yellow onion
- 1 cup diced carrots
- 4 minced garlic cloves
- 5 cups low-sodium chicken broth
- 1 can diced tomatoes
- 1 cup farro
- 1 tsp dried oregano
- Salt to taste
- 1 bay leaf
- ½ cup parsley sprigs with stems included
- 4 cups chopped kale with ribs removed
- 15 oz can of cannellini beans
- ½ cup crumbled feta cheese
- 1 tbsp fresh lemon juice

Instructions:

1. Heat oil in a large pot over medium to high heat.
2. Add celery, carrots, and onions and sauté for 3 minutes. Add garlic and sauté for 30 more seconds.
3. Stir in vegetable broth, tomatoes, oregano, farro, bay leaf, and season with salt to your liking.
4. Add parsley to the soup and bring soup to a boil.
5. Reduce heat just below the medium, cover and let simmer for 20 minutes. Remove parsley, stir in kale and cook 10-15 minutes longer so both farro and kale become tender.
6. Add the cannellini beans and heat for 1 minute.
7. Remove the bay leaf and discard. Stir in the lemon juice and add in additional broth to thin the soup to your liking.
8. Top with feta cheese and serve warm.

Tuscan Soup

Total Time: 35 minutes

Servings: 5

Nutrition Facts:

Calories: 171 kcal

Total Fats: 6 g

Proteins: 7 g

Carbohydrates: 24 g

Ingredients:

- 2 tbsp olive oil
- 1-½ tbsp minced fresh garlic
- 1 cup diced white onion
- 2 tbsp land spice and seasoning blend
- 1 diced celery stalk
- 1 chopped medium zucchini
- 1 large chopped carrot
- 15 oz can of cannellini beans
- 14.5 oz can of diced tomatoes
- 3 tbsp tomato paste (This is optional but will make your broth creamier)
- 6 cups low-sodium vegetable broth
- ⅓ cup chopped fresh basil
- 3 cups chopped spinach
- Sea salt and black pepper to taste

Instructions:

1. Add oil to a pot and put on medium heat. Sauté garlic and onions until onions turn slightly translucent and brown, which takes about 3 minutes.
2. Sprinkle in land spice and seasoning blend and celery. Cook for about 1 minute.

3. Increase heat to high and then add in remaining ingredients and bring to a simmer.
4. Add a pinch of salt and pepper and then reduce heat to low. Place cover and cook on low heat for 30 minutes.
5. Season with sea salt and pepper to your taste and enjoy.

Slow-Cooker Mediterranean Stew

Total Time: 6 hours 45 minutes

Servings: 6

Nutrition Facts:

Calories: 191 kcal

Total Fats: 7.8 g

Proteins: 5.7 g

Carbohydrates: 22.9 g

Ingredients:

- 2-14 oz cans of fire-roasted diced tomatoes, no salt added
- 3 cups low-sodium vegetable broth
- 1 cup chopped onion, coarsely chopped
- ¾ cup of chopped carrots
- 4 minced garlic cloves
- 1 tsp dried oregano
- ½ tsp crushed red pepper
- ¼ tsp ground pepper
- ¾ tsp salt
- 15 oz can of chickpeas, no salt added
- 1 bunch kale with stems, chopped
- 1 tbsp lemon juice
- Fresh basil leaves
- 3 tbsp extra virgin olive oil

- 6 lemon wedges for serving, optional

Instructions:

1. In a 4-quart slow cooker, place the tomatoes, broth, onions, carrots, garlic, oregano, salt, crushed red pepper, and black pepper. Reduce to low heat, place cover, and cook for 6 hours.
2. Take out ¼ cup of liquid from slow cooker and place it into a small bowl.
3. Add 2 tbsp chickpeas and mash with a fork until smooth.
4. Add the mashed chickpeas, the remainder of whole chickpeas, kale, and lemon juice into the slow cooker. Combine everything, then place cover and cook for 30 minutes on low heat or until kale is tender.
5. Divide the stew between 6 bowls and drizzle with olive oil.
6. Garnish with basil and serve with lemon wedges.

Baked Shrimp Stew in Chunky Tomato Sauce

Total Time: 35 minutes

Servings: 6 to 8

Nutrition Facts:

Calories: 377 kcal

Total Fats: 20 g

Proteins: 41.8 g

Carbohydrates: 11.5 g

Ingredients:

- Extra virgin olive oil
- 1 large chopped red onion
- 1 chopped and cored bell pepper
- 1 chopped garlic clove

- 1 tsp sumac
- 1-½ tsp ground coriander
- 1 tsp cumin
- 1 tsp red pepper flakes
- ½ tsp ground green cardamom
- 2, 15 oz cans of diced tomatoes
- Kosher salt and black pepper to taste
- ½ cup of regular water
- 2-½ pound of large shrimp
- 1 cup chopped parsley leaves
- ¼ cup toasted sesame seeds
- ⅓ cup toasted pine nuts
- Lemon wedges to serve, may use lime

Instructions:

1. Turn on the oven to preheat to 375 degrees-F. Position one of the oven racks in the middle.
2. Heat 2 tbsp olive oil on medium heat in a large skillet until it is shimmering but not smoking. Add bell peppers, chopped onions, and garlic. Cook 3-4 minutes and toss regularly.
3. Stir in spices and cook another minute until it is fragrant.
4. Add water and diced tomatoes. Season with kosher salt and pepper to your taste.
5. Bring sauce to a boil, then reduce to a simmer for 10-15 minutes on lower heat.
6. Transfer sauce to a dish that is safe for the oven. Stir shrimp thoroughly into the sauce. Add pine nuts, parsley, and toasted sesame seeds. Cover tightly with foil.
7. Transfer the dish to the oven and bake for about 7 minutes. Uncover and broil briefly until shrimp is ready. Shrimp will be a translucent pink in the thick parts.
8. It is now ready to serve.

Mediterranean Beef Stew

Total Time: 1 hour 45 minutes

Serving: 6

Nutrition Facts:

Calories: 251 kcal

Total fats: 7.7 g

Proteins: 27.2 g

Carbohydrates: 12.4 g

Ingredients:

- 1 ½ tsp olive oil
- 1 ½ pound beef stew meat cut into small pieces, about 1 inch.
- 3 ½ cups halved mushrooms
- 1 ½ cup chopped onions
- 2 cups diagonally sliced carrots
- 1 ½ cups sliced celery
- 1 ½ cups water
- 1 cup dry red wine
- 1 ¼ tsp kosher salt
- ¼ tsp fresh ground black pepper
- ½ tsp thyme
- 1 cans of no-salt-added stewed tomatoes
- 2 bay leaves
- 2 ¼ ounce can of sliced black olives, ripe
- 1 tbsp red wine vinegar
- ¼ cup chopped fresh flat-leaf parsley

Instructions:

1. In a dutch oven, heat oil over medium to high heat.
2. Add beef and cook for 5 minutes until all sides are brown. Remove beef from the pan.
3. Add in carrots, mushrooms, celery, onions, and garlic. Cook for 5 minutes while stirring occasionally.
4. Return beef to the pan.

5. Stir in the water, and the remainder of the ingredients, save for the red wine vinegar, olives, and parsley. Heat until boiling.
6. Reduce to low heat. Cover and let simmer for 1 hour.
7. Stir in olives and cook until beef is tender. Which will take 30 minutes.
8. Take out and discard bay leaves.
9. Stir in the red wine vinegar and sprinkle with parsley. It is ready to serve.

Tomato Stew With Calamari

Total Time: 20 minutes

Servings: 2

Nutrition Facts:

Calories: 416 kcal

Total Fat: 18 g

Proteins: 39 g

Carbohydrates: 19 g

Ingredients:

- 3 minced garlic cloves
- 1 red onion cut into rings
- 2 tbsp olive oil
- 14 oz can of whole peeled tomatoes
- 1 regular tomatoes, cut into cubes
- 1 pound squid, cleaned
- 1 tsp fresh parsley
- ½ tsp rosemary
- 1 tsp fresh dill
- Salt to taste
- Fresh ground black pepper to taste

Instructions:

1. Heat the olive oil on medium heat in a saucepan. Add in garlic and onions. Cook until the onions are translucent.
2. Add the canned tomatoes. Fill the empty can with water and also pour into the pan. Let simmer for a few minutes.
3. Slice the squid into rings, then add the squid and tomatoes to the tomato sauce you just made. Simmer for 5 minutes or until the squid is cooked.
4. Sprinkle with the salt and pepper for flavoring.
5. Finely chop all of the herbs and add them to the soup. It is now ready to serve.

These are just some of the popular dishes from the various countries surrounding the Mediterranean Sea. Of course, with the many common ingredients, you will have a lot of creative liberty in making your own phenomenal dishes. Just make sure to stick with the measurements and similar food groups and you will be able to produce a number of delicious and healthy meals for you and your friends or family.

I compiled these recipes in a way so they would be as diverse as possible to satisfy even the pickiest palate palates. But you can't really go wrong when there are so many great dishes to choose from.

Notes:

Chapter 4: Delicious Drinks

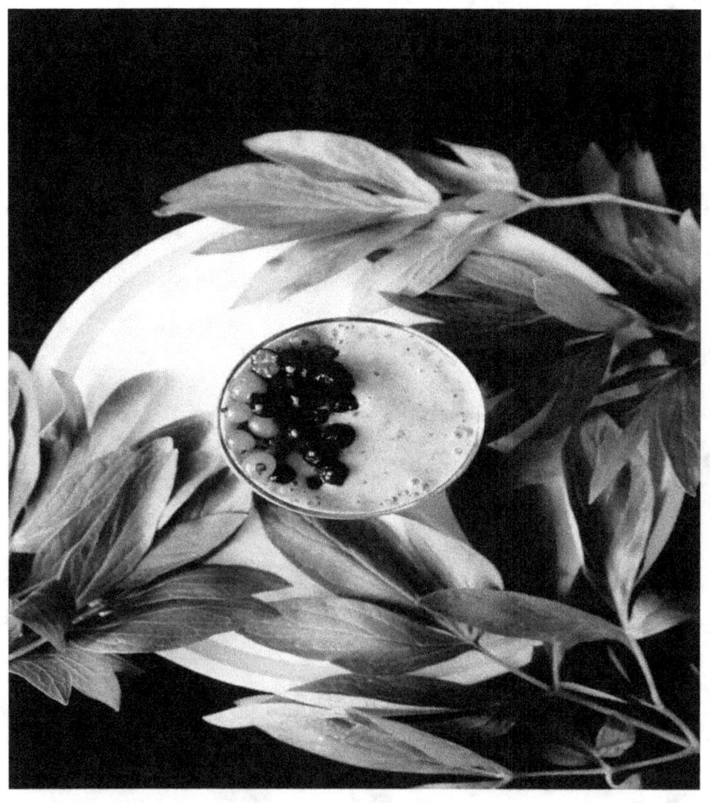

We have provided multiple diverse recipes for delicious meal plans that are part of the Mediterranean diet. We will now provide recipes for some delicious drinks. These drinks can complement a particular meal, or be meals in themselves. With the rich amount of nutrients present, they are bound to fill you up. Before you begin making these smoothies, make sure you have a reliable blender as you will be using it often. These smoothies are very easy to make and take no time so they are perfect for those days when you just can't get ahead of the clock but want something yummy.

Smoothies

Anti-Inflammatory Blueberry Smoothie

Total Time: 5 minutes

Servings: 1

Nutrition Facts:

Calories: 340 kcal

Total Fats: 13 g

Proteins: 9 g

Carbohydrates: 55 g

Ingredients:

- 1 frozen banana
- 1 cup frozen blueberries
- 2 handfuls spinach or other leafy greens
- 1 cup almond milk
- 1 tbsp almond butter
- ¼ tsp cinnamon
- ¼ tsp cayenne pepper (Add according to your own spice level)
- 1 tsp maca powder

Instructions:

1. Combine all of the ingredients in a high-powered blender and blend until smooth. Presto!

Mediterranean Smoothie

Total Time: 5 Minutes

Servings: 1

Nutrition Facts:

Calories: 168 kcal

Total fats: 1 g

Proteins: 4 g

Carbohydrates: 39 g

Ingredients:

- 2 cups of loosely packed baby green spinach
- 1 tsp minced ginger root
- 1 pre sliced frozen banana
- 1 small mango
- ½ cup beet juice
- ½ cup skim milk
- 6 ice cubes

Instructions:

1. Toss all of the ingredients in a high-powered blender and blend until smooth. It is ready to serve immediately.

Pick Me Up Breakfast Smoothie

Total Time: 5 minutes

Servings: 1

Nutrition Facts:

Calories: 297 kcal

Total fats: 4 g

Proteins: 6 g

Carbohydrates: 66 g

Ingredients:

- 1 tbsp ground flax seed
- 4 fresh strawberries
- 6 oz coconut water, may also use plain water
- 6 baby spinach leaves

- 1 whole banana

Instructions:

1. Place ingredients in a blender and blend until smooth, about one minute or desired thickness. It is ready to serve.

Superfoods Smoothie

Total Time: 5 minutes

Servings: 3

Nutrition Facts:

Calories: 131 kcal

Total Fats: 1 g

Proteins: 7 g

Carbohydrates: 26 g

Ingredients:

- 1 frozen banana, sliced
- 1 cup of frozen berries, unsweetened
- 1 cup baby spinach, loosely packed
- ½ inch slice of ginger root
- ½ cup of Greek yogurt
- 1 cup of chilled green tea
- ½ cup of pure pomegranate juice
- 1 cup crushed ice

Instructions:

1. Place all of the ingredients in a blender and blend until desired consistency.
2. For a thinner smoothie, you may add some more green tea to your liking.
3. It is now ready to serve.

Immune Booster Smoothie

Total Time: 5 minutes

Servings: 1

Nutrition Facts:

Calories: 156 kcal

Total Fats: 3 g

Proteins: 10 g

Carbohydrates: 26 g

Ingredients:

- 1 frozen pre sliced banana
- 1 ginger root, about half an inch
- ⅛ tsp cinnamon
- ½ peeled avocado
- 1 cup red kale
- ¼ cup coconut meat fresh from the coconut is best
- 1 cup baby spinach
- 1 cup frozen red grapes or blueberries
- ¼ cup pomegranate seeds
- 1 ½ cup chilled green tea, unsweetened

Instructions:

1. Place all of the ingredients in a blender, about a minute until smooth.
2. Add green tea for a thinner smoothie, add ice for a thicker smoothie. It is now ready to serve.

This may be one of the healthiest smoothies you can make.

Cleanse And Detox Smoothie

Total Time: 5 minutes

Servings: 1

Nutrition Facts:

Calories: 194 kcal

Total Fats: 6.2 g

Proteins: 5.5 g

Carbohydrates: 34.1 g

Ingredients:

- Juice from 1 lemon
- 1 cup kale
- 1 organic apple
- 1 rib of celery
- ⅓ cup flat parsley leaves
- 1 tbsp ground flax seeds or chia seeds
- ¼ tsp ground cinnamon
- 1 ¼ cup of regular water

Instructions:

- Add all of the ingredients into a blender and blend until smooth.
- Pour over ice and it is ready to serve.

Peanut Butter and Banana Smoothie

Total Time: 5 minutes

Servings: 2

Nutrition Facts:

Calories: 173 kcal

Total Fats: 6 g

Proteins: 12 g

Carbohydrates: 20 g

Ingredients:

- 1 scoop of your favorite protein powder
- 1 ½ cup of almond milk
- 1 pre sliced frozen banana
- 1 tbsp peanut butter

Instructions:

1. Place all of the ingredients in a high-powered blender and blend until smooth. It is now ready to serve, and share!

If you love peanut butter, you will love this smoothie.

Wild Blueberry, Mint, and Flaxseed Smoothie

Total Time: 5 minutes

Servings: 2

Nutrition Facts:

Calories: 200 kcal

Total fats: 7 g

Proteins: 10 g

Carbohydrates: 26 g

Ingredients:

- 2 cups chilled almond milk
- ¼ cup frozen blueberries
- 2 cups chilled almond milk
- 1 tbsp raw honey
- 2 fresh mint leaves

Instructions:

1. You may be seeing a pattern here by now. Wash and place all ingredients in a blender until smooth.
2. Ready to serve.

Kale-Pineapple Smoothie

Total Time: 5 minutes

Servings: 2

Nutrition Facts:

Calories: 140 kcal

Total Fats: 2.5 g

Proteins: 4 g

Carbohydrates: 30 g

Ingredients:

- 1 Persian cucumber chopped
- Fresh mint
- 1 tbsp honey
- 1 cup coconut milk
- 1-½ cups pineapple pieces
- ¼ pound kale

Instructions:

1. Gather all of the ingredients and wash thoroughly.
2. Place in a blender and blend on high speed until smooth.
3. Serve!

Juices

Along with smoothies, the Mediterranean diet boasts many tasty and healthy juices as well. These fresh juice recipes will be a compliment to almost any meal. Unfortunately, people assume that store bought juices are healthy options. However, these contain high amounts of added sugar and other substances that deplete the nutritional value. Sodas are also not a healthy option. In addition, many other drinks that are represented as healthy are anything but that. Fresh juices like the ones we will discuss are the best things to drink. If you are getting sick of water, try out these Mediterranean juices.

Simple Green Juice

Total Time: 15 minutes

Servings: 2 large glasses

Nutrition Facts:

Calories: 92 kcal

Total fats: 0.8 g

Proteins: 2.8 g

Carbohydrates: 21 g

Ingredients:

- 1 bunch of kale
- 1 inch piece of peeled fresh ginger
- 1 large apple
- ½ large English cucumber
- 5 celery stalks with the ends trimmed
- 1 oz fresh parsley

Instructions:

1. Wash all of the vegetables thoroughly.
2. Place all of the ingredients in a blender on high until smooth.
3. Ready to serve!

Good Digestion Celery Juice

Total Time: 50 minutes

Servings: 2

Nutrition Facts:

Calories: 95 kcal

Total Fats: 1.1 g

Proteins: 2.9 g

Carbohydrates: 21 g

Ingredients:

- 2 pounds of chopped organic celery
- 2 large chopped cucumbers
- 1 large naval orange
- ½ lemon

Instructions:

1. Soak all ingredients in a bath of apple cider vinegar and water for 15 minutes. Ratio about ½ cup vinegar to 1-gallon water.
2. Place all of the ingredients in a high-powered blender and blend until smooth.

Detoxifying Beet Juice

Total Time: 15 minutes

Servings: 4

Nutrition Facts:

Calories: 83 kcal

Total Fats: 0.1 g

Proteins: 1.3 g

Carbohydrates: 21.9 g

Ingredients:

- 1 pound of beets with the end cut off and washed
- 2 pounds of chopped carrots
- 1 bunch of celery
- Juice from 2 full lemons
- Juice from 1 full lime

- 1 bunch of flat-leaf parsley
- 1 chopped red apple

Instructions:

1. Make sure produce is clean before chopping. Cut into small enough pieces to fit into the feeder of your juicer.
2. Feed the vegetables a little bit at a time into your juicer, alternating between harder and softer textured fruits.

Carrot Apple Celery Ginger Juice

Total Time: 10 minutes

Servings: 4

Nutrition Facts:

Calories: 121 kcal

Total fats: 1 g

Proteins: 1 g

Carbohydrates: 30 g

Ingredients:

- 14 oz carrot
- 14 oz apple
- ½ oz ginger
- 2 oz celery
- 2 tbsp sugar
- 8 oz ice cubes

Instructions:

1. Wash all of the produce with water.
2. Peel and cut the carrots into quarters vertically. Peel the apple and cut them into small chunks. Chop the celery and scrape off the skin of the ginger.

3. Run all of the ingredients a little bit at a time through the juicer. Whatever your juicer can handle.
4. Stir the juice and divide evenly between 4 glasses.

Celery Ginger Juice

Total Time: 5 minutes

Servings: 1

Nutrition Facts:

Calories: 154 kcal

Total fats: 0

Proteins:2 g

Carbohydrates: 41 g

Ingredients:

- 1 bunch celery chopped
- ½ English cucumber cut into quarters
- 1 large green apple cut into smaller pieces
- ½ lemon
- 1 inch knob of ginger

Instructions:

1. After washing, run celery and cucumber through a juicer on a low setting.
2. Switch to a high setting and juice the apple, lemon, and ginger.
3. Pour into a glass and it's ready to serve.

Mediterranean-Style Mint Lemonade

Total Time: 10

Servings: 5

Nutrition Facts:

Calories: 180 kcal

Total Fats: 0

Proteins: 1 g

Carbohydrates: 49 g

Ingredients:

- 2 cups water
- Juice from 1 lemon
- 2 cups ice, crushed
- 2 large lemons
- 1 bunch fresh mint leaves with stems removed
- 1 cup sugar, may add more to your liking but still be mindful of sugar intake

Instructions:

1. Before starting, peel the large lemons and cut into small pieces so they will blend easily.
2. Take all of the ingredients and add them to your blender. The more high-quality, the better.
3. Blend on high-speed and liquefy the ingredients. There may be small strands of solids still remaining.
4. You may add more mint-leaves or sugar to your desired taste.
5. Pour the contents into a pitcher through a strainer to catch any remaining solids.
6. Refrigerate until it is ready to serve.

Not only is the Mediterranean diet home to many great foods but also many great drinks. We hope that you will enjoy some of these flavors to compliment your meals. Just like with the cuisines, you can get creative with these drink recipes as well. Look at what various fruits and vegetables you can combine according to your taste buds and feel free to mix them to make your own delicious juices. Really, if you can imagine the fruit or vegetable, you can somehow make a juice out of it. Some things to consider when creating a juice from various ingredients are the taste, nutrition content and water/liquid content. The above juices were just examples. There are a few fruits and vegetables you want to consider as being the best as far as making high-quality juices.

- Kale
- Carrots
- Beets
- Celery
- Tomatoes
- Wheatgrass
- Cucumber
- Parsley
- Oranges
- Apples
- Berries
- Broccoli
- Ginger
- Cabbage

Nutrient-dense smoothies and juices are common in the Mediterranean diet plan. Other acceptable drinks are various teas like green tea, lavender tea, lemon tea, and herbal tea. In addition, regular black coffee with minimal or zero sugar is fine. We recommend using raw honey as a sweetener rather than sugar whenever possible. Adding turmeric or cinnamon to coffee has also become a popular thing to do. Turmeric complements the aroma of coffee quite well. Finally, pure water is always the most acceptable drink to accompany every meal. Unhealthy drinks cause the same issues as meals, so be careful with what you are regularly drinking.

Notes:

Chapter 5: Making The Transition

Now that I have thoroughly engaged you with the information and recipes needed to take hold of the Mediterranean diet, it is time for you to make the transition. I hope the previous chapters have excited you and you are ready to start incorporating these food choices into your life. I am here to help you make the switch as efficiently as possible. I am providing you with a 21-day meal plan that will keep you inspired and help hold yourself accountable for making it happen.

Sample Schedule

Monday:

- Breakfast: Bacon and eggs, coffee with cream and sugar
- Snack: Cookies
- Lunch: Pizza and soda
- Snack: chips
- Dinner: Falafel sandwich

Tuesday:

- Breakfast: Shakshuka
- Snack: Cookies
- Lunch: Hamburger and fries
- Snack: Handful of almonds
- Dinner: Mediterranean chicken

Wednesday:

- Breakfast: Blueberry oatmeal, banana, and green tea
- Snack: Chocolate bar
- Lunch: Greek salad with grilled chicken
- Snack: Handful of walnuts
- Dinner: Lamb kabob

Thursday:

- Breakfast: Spinach and egg whites with black coffee
- Snack: Handful of almonds
- Lunch: Falafel salad
- Snack: Greek yogurt
- Dinner: Lemon and lime grilled chicken

Friday:

- Breakfast: Oatmeal with raw honey and green tea
- Snack: Celery sticks
- Lunch: Grilled chicken pita
- Snack: Handful of almonds and pita chips
- Dinner: Greek salad, roasted potatoes.

With this sample schedule, I have you slowly transitioned into the full Mediterranean diet by day five. This will allow your body to naturally adjust, rather than make a major shift overnight. It is recommended to have a transitional period before fully committing to a major diet plan.

The 21-Day Plan

I will now go over a thorough and well-designed 21-day action plan that will help you make the transition to full time Mediterranean dieter. The keyword here is "action" because if you don't act, this part of the book will be useless to you. If this sounds harsh, we certainly don't mean it to be. We simply want you to understand just how vital it is to stay the course once we get this plan started. During this 21-day plan, there will be no room for wavering. This means, if you fall out of the plan and have a slip-up, you must start over. This is because it takes a minimum of 21 days to develop a strong habit. We want you to be fully committed for 21 days and if you can do that, then you will have some time to celebrate and have a few cheat days.

After the 21-day plan has been achieved, our expectation is that you will have fully incorporated the diet into your life and habitually eat the traditional cuisines on a regular basis. Once you have developed this habit, having a cheat day here or there will not affect you. As long as they are few and far between. You may be wondering what the significance of 21 days is? Much research shows that it takes a minimum of 21 days to develop a habit. For some it's more, for others less, but this is usually the average. Once you have developed the habit, it becomes ingrained in you and much harder to break.

With the Mediterranean diet, as long as you stick to the ingredients, you don't really have to worry about specific portion sizes, calorie counting, or keeping track of nutrients. The diet plan is a little more liberal in that manner. Being as nutrient-dense as the food is, you will have very little issues getting the substances your body needs. We want you to eat and feel satiated. Once you feel full, you may stop eating for the time being. We certainly do not want you to overeat. Also, be mindful that even though healthy fats like olive oil, nuts, and avocados are utilized, eating them in excess can still cause fat to settle in hard to reach areas, like the waistline. Also, we recommend no large meals prior to sleeping. This can disrupt your sleep patterns. We have provided various recipes, ingredients, and food groups to be used in the Mediterranean diet earlier in this book. Follow these recipes and feel free to develop your own with the various ingredients.

For those who are quite new to the Mediterranean diet, and we will assume that the majority of you are, here is a short guideline you can follow when determining your daily meal plans. Again, calorie counting, nutrient tracking, and portion sizes can vary with each person. It is not critical to keep track of these religiously. However, we hope this shortlist is helpful in getting you started.

Recommended Servings

- Vegetable: About three servings a day. One serving equals ½ cup cooked and 1 cup of raw vegetables.
- Fruits: Also about three servings per day. Berries are often the most recommended types of fruit.
- Olive Oil: Up to four tablespoons a day. This includes what it used for cooking.
- Legumes: Three servings per week. Legumes can include various beans, peas, alfalfa, cashews, and peanuts.
- Fish: Three servings a week. Fishes with high omega-3 fatty acids are recommended. Fish is a major source of protein in the Mediterranean diet plan.
- Nuts: Three servings per week. One serving equals ¼ cup. Raw and unsalted nuts are the best option.
- Starches: Three to six servings a day. Starches include barley, whole grains, brown rice, potatoes, and quinoa.
- White meat: Three servings per week. A serving is about three ounces. Skinless poultry is recommended over red meat. Poultry includes chicken, turkey, pheasant, and ostrich.
- Red Meat: One serving a week and make sure it is lean meat.
- Dairy/Eggs: Three servings per week. Low-fat options on milk, yogurt, and cottage cheese are recommended. There are no limits to eggs. The fat and cholesterol in the egg yolk is not really enough to create problems.
- Desserts: One serving per week. If possible, let fruit be your dessert. Of course, it is certainly okay to indulge once in a while. Also, we recommend desserts with healthier ingredients and smaller portions. Baklava, for example, is a better option than triple-chocolate cake.

- Wine: If you enjoy wine, we recommend four to 6 ounces a day. We do not recommend beer or other hard liquors with the Mediterranean diet.

We hope that you have a good understanding of what the Mediterranean diet is by this point. If you are ready to get started with the 21-day plan, then let's go!

Day 1

By day one, you should be fully committed to the diet plan.

- Breakfast: Egg white omelet with oatmeal with blueberries on top. A good drink choice is a black coffee, green tea, or plain water.
- Mid-morning snack: A handful of almonds.
- Lunch: Falafel pita that also includes tomatoes, onions, black olives, lettuce, and yogurt sauce. An eight-ounce glass of water.
- Mid-day snack: Pita chips with hummus dip.
- Dinner: Grilled lemon chicken with a glass of water.
- Late night snack: Greek yogurt. A late-night snack shortly before going to bed is recommended to prevent you from getting hungry overnight. It also keeps your metabolism going. Something like Greek yogurt, cottage cheese, plain yogurt, or a small piece of fruit is recommended.

Day 2

- Breakfast: Bowl of oatmeal with bananas and raw honey on top. Black coffee with a small amount of raw honey for sweetener.
- Mid-morning snack: ½ cup of blueberries.
- Lunch: Greek salad with grilled chicken and a glass of water.
- Mid-day snack: 1 cup of strawberries.
- Dinner: Lean steak strips with roasted potatoes. Red wine for drinking.

- Late night snack: Apple slices.

Day 3

- Breakfast: Egg white omelet with spinach, tomatoes, black pepper, and basil. Black coffee with raw honey.
- Mid-morning snack: Banana.
- Lunch: Mediterranean pizza with feta cheese, apple slices, and an 8-ounce glass of water.
- Mid-day snack: Carrot sticks with hummus.
- Dinner: Ratatouille with a glass of wine.
- Late-night snack: Blueberry Greek yogurt.

Day 4

- Breakfast: Loaded omelet with bell pepper, feta cheese, tomatoes, black pepper, and basil. Green tea for drinking.
- Mid-morning snack: Handful of almonds.
- Lunch: Grilled chicken pita with lettuce, tomatoes, onions, and olives. Blueberry smoothie for drinking.
- Mid-day snack: Handful of cashews.
- Dinner: Chicken Shawarma with brown rice and a side of quinoa. 8-ounce glass of water for drinking.
- Late-night snack: Cottage cheese with ground black pepper.

Day 5

- Breakfast: Breakfast smoothie with apples, kale, lemon, blueberries, and celery. Plus, a bowl of oatmeal with raw honey.
- Mid-morning snack: A cup of strawberries with Greek yogurt.
- Lunch: Plain Greek salad with a side of pita bread and hummus. An 8-ounce glass of water for drinking.
- Mid-day snack: One banana.

- Dinner: Baked salmon with a side of asparagus and fresh-squeezed orange juice.
- Late-night snack: Apple slices.

Day 6

- Breakfast: Whole wheat toast with a light spread of butter, and a bowl of Greek yogurt with granola, strawberries and raw honey. Green tea for drinking.
- Mid-morning snack: Cup of black coffee with raw honey.
- Lunch: Grilled chicken breast with a small side salad. An 8-ounce glass of water for drinking.
- Mid-day snack: Handful of raspberries.
- Dinner: Lebanese rice with lentils and a side of chickpeas.
- Late-night snack: Plain yogurt with half of a banana.

Day 7

- Breakfast: Egg white omelet with basils and spinach, whole-wheat toast, and black coffee with raw honey.
- Mid-morning snack: Handful of peanuts.
- Lunch: Falafel salad with an 8-ounce glass of water.
- Mid-day snack: One apple.
- Dinner: Baked cod with lemon and garlic. One glass of wine for drinking.
- Late-night snack: Carrot sticks with hummus.

We have officially finished the first week of the plan. Assess yourself and how you are feeling. You should notice a marked increase in digestion, energy, productivity, and your overall sense of well-being. Also, look back on the past seven days and determine if you stuck to the Mediterranean diet all the way. Remember, our expectation is that you follow this plan completely. If you did not, then please start over. We make this plan simple, but not easy.

Day 8

Breakfast: Green tea, breakfast couscous, oatmeal, and a banana.

Mid-morning snack: Greek yogurt.

Lunch: Vegetable soup, grilled chicken and broccoli.

Mid-day snack: Cup of raspberries.

Dinner: Baked salmon, ratatouille.

Late-night snack: Plain yogurt with raisins

Day 9

Breakfast: Oatmeal with a morning smoothie.

Mid-morning snack: Apple slices.

Lunch: Falafel sandwich with green juice.

Mid-day snack: Unsalted peanuts.

Dinner: Greek baked meatballs with bread on the side.

Late-night snack: Cottage cheese with black olives.

Day 10

Breakfast: Shakshuka with water.

Mid-morning snack: Carrot sticks.

Lunch: Greek lemon rice with carrots and potatoes.

Mid-day snack: 1 cup of blueberries.

Dinner: Mediterranean grilled chicken.

Late-night snack: Banana.

Day 11

Breakfast: Scrambled eggs with turmeric, black pepper, tomatoes and bell peppers. Black coffee

Mid-morning snack: Half of a blueberry smoothie.

Lunch: Spicy Mediterranean pasta, with pomegranate juice, fresh.

Mid-day snack: Other half of blueberry smoothie.

Dinner: Mediterranean calamari with fresh squeezed orange juice.

Late-night snack: Greek yogurt.

Day 12

Breakfast: Oatmeal topped with blueberries, raw honey, and almonds, with a green tea.

Mid-morning snack: Handful of walnuts.

Lunch: Lebanese rice, roasted tomatoes with a glass of water for drinking.

Mid-day snack: Handful of almonds.

Dinner: Mediterranean pizza.

Late-night snack: Vanilla Greek yogurt.

Day 13

Breakfast: Mediterranean breakfast burrito with a cup of black coffee.

Mid-morning snack: Fresh-squeezed apple/kale/spinach juice.

Lunch: Mediterranean orzo salad with grilled chicken.

Mid-day snack: Celery sticks.

Dinner: Mediterranean lamb shanks with fresh green juice.

Late-night snack: Handful of grapes.

Day 14

Breakfast: Egg Muffins with green tea and a breakfast smoothie.

Mid-morning snack: Apple slices with almond butter.

Lunch: Easy Italian baked chicken with Mediterranean style mint lemonade.

Mid-day snack: Baby carrots with hummus.

Dinner: Cup of mixed berries.

We have officially made it past two weeks. How did you do? Did you make it through without faltering? We hope so, because if you didn't, please start over. We also hope you are starting to feel better overall. Remember, adjust these foods accordingly as you please because there are several Mediterranean meal options. Let's keep going and finish out this last week strong. Remember, not only is this a plan, but also a challenge.

Day 15

Breakfast: Let's mix it up here. Oatmeal, blueberries, 2 egg muffins, apple slices and water.

Mid-morning snack: Orange

Lunch: Mediterranean chicken with green olives and beets juice.

Mid-day snack: Pecans.

Dinner: Braised lamb shanks with grapefruit jicama green juice.

Late-night snack: Cottage cheese with black pepper and red pepper.

Day 16

Breakfast: Egg white omelet with oregano and spinach. Coffee with raw honey.

Mid-morning snack: Raisins

Lunch: Chickpea salad with pita bread and hummus. Glass of water for drinking.

Mid-day snack: More pita bread with hummus.

Dinner: Roasted potatoes with cauliflower rice. Green juice for drinking.

Late-night snack: Carrots with hummus.

Day 17

Breakfast: Breakfast smoothie with a banana.

Mid-morning snack: Greek yogurt with whole grain granola.

Lunch: Mediterranean cod with asparagus.

Mid-day snack: Mixed berries.

Dinner: Lean steak strips over long grain rice with lemon and pepper.

Late-night snack: Almonds

Day 18

Breakfast: Breakfast couscous with green tea.

Mid-morning snack: Apple slices.

Lunch: Grilled chicken gyro with a yogurt drink.

Mid-day snack: Blueberries

Dinner: Mediterranean snapper with cooked carrots.

Late-night snack: Strawberries.

Day 19

Breakfast: Mediterranean breakfast sandwich with an almond milk for drinking.

Mid-morning snack: Banana.

Lunch: Fattoush salad with falafel on the side.

Mid-day snack: Small couscous salad.

Dinner: Mediterranean chicken with tomatoes and broccoli.

Late-night snack: Small tabouli salad.

Day 20

Breakfast: Superfood smoothie, apple slices, and blueberries.

Mid-morning snack: Banana.

Lunch: Mediterranean stew with pita and hummus as a side.

Mid-day snack: Falafel patties.

Dinner: Mediterranean steak bowl.

Late-night snack: Greek yogurt with strawberries.

Day 21 Final Day!

Breakfast: Immune booster smoothie, banana and a green tea.

Mid-morning snack: Plain yogurt with black olive and peppers.

Lunch: Large Greek salad with grilled chicken

Mid-day snack: Small Mediterranean potato salad.

Dinner: Lebanese rice with lentils and rustic roasted potatoes.

Late-night snack: Cottage cheese with black olives and pepper.

Congratulations! You have finished the 21-day Mediterranean diet meal plan. Feel good about yourself because challenges like these are not easy. We hope that you have developed some great eating habits at this point and were able to follow the plan all the way to the end. If for some reason you could not make it the 21-days and still want to continue, then we advise you start over and really complete 21 days straight. The reason we are so adamant about this is because we want you to really develop the habit of eating right, and you cannot do this if you don't challenge yourself and remain motivated. For 21-days, we want you to fully embrace this diet plan and see how it makes you feel.

Of course, this meal plan is just an example. You can use this one, or also develop your own. The main things to remember are sticking to the Mediterranean diet plan and going 21 days without faltering. If you falter, you must start over. Before you partake in this challenge, we recommend incorporating the diet into your life slowly, so you get used to it.

One thing that the Mediterranean region promotes, that is missing in much of the Western world, is using mealtime to break away from the daily grind. Essentially, during meals, families gather and spend time mingling with each other. They turn off the television and get rid of any other distractions that take away from the moment of the meal. People don't just scarf down a salad or yogurt while reading emails. They take the time to sit and enjoy the meals they are eating. In this manner, the Mediterranean becomes a lifestyle. If you are able to incorporate this into your lifestyle, we highly recommend it. Even minor changes like eating dinner at the dinner table rather than in front of the television are good steps.

Notes:

Chapter 6: To Your Success

We hope that the information in this book finds you well. We went over many aspects of the Mediterranean diet, but our goal was for you to understand everything that it encompasses, including all of the health benefits. Eating these nutrient-rich foods on a regular basis will be quite beneficial for your health and when you couple it with a healthy lifestyle, you will experience a tremendous increase in your quality of life. We want to make sure this happens for you so we are here to provide as much encouragement and guidance as we can.

The first thing to understand is that making a transition takes time. Good habits take a while to develop so don't be too hard on yourself when you are making the necessary changes to your diet. Start slow and take baby steps each day. If you try to completely overhaul your diet overnight, the chances of you succeeding are quite low. You will likely revert right back to your old eating habits because your body did not have time to adjust accordingly. Our bodies are much more intelligent than we give them credit for.

Consider these steps to building new habits:

- Start with a very small habit that you can accomplish easily and don't need any motivation to do. For example, incorporate one type of Mediterranean cuisine into your diet plan on day one. This can be done with minimal effort and is as simple as eating a piece of fruit as a snack rather than a bag of chips.
- Increase your habit in very small ways on a daily basis. If you start eating one type of Mediterranean cuisine on day one, eat two the next day. Or, eat one for several days until you can work up to two. Whatever is easier for you to build up this habit. The more that our old habits are ingrained in us, the longer it may take to readjust.

- Break habits into smaller pieces. When starting out, if you eat 2 different Mediterranean cuisines one day, the next day eat one and then go back up to two. Do this until you are able to eat two every day and then continue to increase from there.
- When you get off track, get back on as quickly as you can. We all have slip-ups; however, it is important not to fall completely off the wagon. Missing a habit once will not really affect your long-term progress. However, missing it day after day will make it impossible for you to form. You don't need to have an all-or-nothing mentality. You just need to be consistent and realize you are not perfect.
- Be patient and stick with a pace that you can sustain. Progress takes time, so be patient with yourself. The goal is to fully incorporate the Mediterranean diet into your life. Save for a few cheat meals, this will become your daily meal plan. The transition may take a while, but it will happen.
- Don't give up! This may be the most important advice there is. Do not give up! It will become difficult at times, but the results will be worth it in the end. Generally, things that are worth it don't come easy.

Many of these steps were covered in the 21-day plan and everything leading up to it. In the sample schedule in the previous chapter, we spoke about how you can incorporate small meals every day into your daily habits. Take baby steps and do not try to make major changes overnight. Especially something that can affect your physiology. Your body will thank you for this. Always remember that a small amount of progress is still progress.

Using The Buddy System

Have you ever needed help with anything? The answer is probably yes, because the truth is, we cannot get through this world on our own. As much as we would like to be independent, we all need someone to help us from time to time. This help can be as simple as giving emotional support. When we go to the gym, many of us have workout partners that complement us, and also hold us accountable. Some people will use a personal trainer. This is all part of using the buddy system. That being said, why not use the same system for your diet?

When developing your new diet plan, reach out to a friend who may also like to join in. Someone who is also looking to improve their health. Or, it can just be someone who you will trust to hold you accountable. Use them as part of your buddy system. While it is ultimately your responsibility what results you obtain, having a backup person giving you support is a major benefit. You can do your part to help them as well.

If you don't want to go at it alone, you won't have to. Reach out to someone and ask them or help. We advise that you don't reach out to your friend who will just be nice to you and tell you what you want to hear. In this situation, it is best to reach out to your most honest and blunt friend. Of course, you also don't want someone who is simply abusive or insulting. Honesty and kindness are a great couple. We hope that the recipes in this book provided you with some motivation as well. we expect that the more you eat the Mediterranean diet, the more you will fall in love with it.

Write It Down

Many self-help and motivational experts will tell you to write things down. Whatever you may feel about their other words, this is definitely sage advice. Writing things down makes them concrete. You are much more likely to follow through on something if it is written down. In the case of the Mediterranean diet, write down exactly what you will eat or have eaten on a particular day and assess how closely you followed through on the diet plan. Furthermore, if you felt good on this day, try to outdo yourself the following day. Writing things down also allows you to look back on the progress you have made. You can use this as motivation to keep moving ahead. Write it down, track it, and hold yourself accountable!

Getting Medical Advice

One thing we want to precaution you of is that everyone reacts differently to different meal plans. Before embarking on a new diet plan like this one, we ask that you receive proper medical advice. The information we provide in this book is not meant to replace medical advice from a professional. Seek out your family physician or other primary healthcare provider and ask for their recommendations.

Now that we have reached the end of this book, we must ask, what is stopping you? This is a serious question. We have addressed the taste issue. You will never lack flavor with this meal plan. We have addressed the tremendous health benefits. What more could you ask for? There are essentially two things stopping people: time and money. People feel that they don't have time to make proper Mediterranean meals. While it is true that much preparation and many ingredients must be used, it does not take as much time as you may think. This was showcased by many of the recipes we provided in the previous chapters. Furthermore, you can make several servings that will last a few days. The various ingredients are readily available nowadays. You don't have to find a specialty store. Your local grocery store will carry so many of these ingredients. Once you get cooking, you will find that it's a lot of fun and you won't mind the time it takes after this.

As far as the issue of money, it is not as expensive as one may think. While I don't claim to know your budget, buying healthy ingredients and creating your own meals, in the long run, will be cheaper than buying food outside every day. Since the ingredients are readily available, you won't have to spend much to get them or order online. As mentioned before, you can create many servings with the ingredients and food groups that are utilized. As you have seen in the recipes, I utilized small amounts of ingredients as well, so they will last you several meals. In addition, the herbs and spices have relatively long shelf-lives. The bottom line, it won't hurt your pocketbook as much as you think. We hope that we have addressed your questions and concerns in this book, and you are now able to fully incorporate the Mediterranean diet plan into your everyday life.

Conclusion

Thank you for taking the time to read *The Mediterranean Diet for Beginners: Practical Guide Step by Step for Beginners to Lose Weight, Be Long-lived and Live in Health, With Simple and Fast Recipes.* I expect that it provided you with a well-rounded understanding of the Mediterranean diet and everything that it encompasses. This will truly provide all of you with a diverse meal plan that will be flavorful and healthy at the same time. Unfortunately, it is difficult to find great tasting food that is also good for you. Furthermore, much of the health food out there is anything but this. Juices that claim to be healthy are loaded with sugar. Meals that claim to have hearty ingredients with fillers and way too much salt.

With the Mediterranean diet, this will not be of concern. If you follow the traditional meal plans with authentic ingredients, we all but guarantee delicious food that will have tremendous health benefits, give you extra energy, and help you prevent many chronic illnesses. It may sound too hard to believe, but in reality, it's not as unlikely as you would think. The dietary content that we ingest plays a significant role in how our bodies function. We get a large number of nutrients from our food. It makes sense then that what we eat produces what we become. When we eat well, our bodies thank us. Next time you are feeling hungry, instead of going for that greasy burger, try a falafel sandwich.

In addition to understanding the Mediterranean diet, we hope that you will fully incorporate it into your lives by following the many recipe plans in this book. These will provide a base for your cooking and allow you to create your own delicious meal ideas as an offshoot. Just be mindful of the ingredients that you use because they are what determine whether your meal is healthy or not.

I want you to succeed and advise you to also try the 21-day plan. Feel free to create your own variations of it as the one I provided is only meant to be used as an example. In the end, I want you to experience a healthy and life-changing diet each day. If you enjoyed this book, I hope you will share the information with many of your friends and family, as it is much more fun to break bread with those you love. The Mediterranean diet is the ultimate healthy diet and I want as many people to experience it as possible.

www.ingramcontent.com/pod-product-compliance
Lightning Source LLC
Chambersburg PA
CBHW070709250726

48662CB00001B/337